Also by Sandy Johnson :

The Cuppi

Walk a Winter Beach

Against the Law

The Book of Elders; Life Stories & Wisdom of Great American Indians

The Book of Tibetan Elders

The Brazilian Healer with the Kitchen Knife

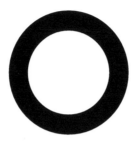

THE THIRTEENTH MOON

· · · · · · · · · · · · ·

a Journey into the Heart of Healing

SANDY JOHNSON

For Mark, Billy, Anthony, Wendy, Sally and Debbie

And in memory of Bill

Sandy Johnson

TABLE OF CONTENTS

• • • • • • • • • • • •

Preface.. 10

January : *The Moon of the Terrible*........................... 26

February : *The Ice Moon*.................................... 38

March : *The Crow Moon*.................................... 50

April : *The Moon of the Awakening*........................... 58

May : *The Moon when Ponies Shed their Shaggy Hair* 72

June : *The Spider Moon*..................................... 84

July : *The Moon of the Sacred Sundance*..................... 94

August : *The Moon of the Joyful*............................ 102

September : *The Moon of Change*............................ 112

October : *The Hunter's Moon*............................... 130

November : *The Thanking Moon*............................ 148

December : *The Turning Moon*............................. 158

The Dark Moon.. 170

The Thirteenth Moon 190

Epilogue... 226

Rise up nimbly

and go on your

strange journey.

Rumi

Preface

· · · · · · · · · · · ·

It is dawn. Three days into the new year of 2006, I am standing at the window of my tenth-floor apartment staring out at the morning moon which is full. On the other side of the building the sun is just beginning to rise; I can see its bright orange reflection on the windows of the buildings across from me. There is a strange, other-worldly quality about this pale morning moon. I can still make out the rabbit (I have never understood why people persist in seeing a man in the moon when it should be clear to anyone that it's a rabbit up there—ears pointing to the right, cottontail bottom at the lower right.) I ponder this rather than think about the phone call that came late yesterday afternoon, twelve hours ago, from my doctor.

New Year's Day was only three days ago. I had my traditional New Year's Day party—champagne, Bloody Marys, and my house special, johnnycakes (small corn cakes topped with a dollop of crème fraiche and red caviar). It felt especially festive. While winter raged across the rest of the country, in Southern California we were enjoying our 70-degree golden days. I had just settled into my new apartment, which I loved so much that I wanted the lease to read: Forever Plus Six Months. Floor-to-ceiling windows face north and west and overlook the hills of Griffith Park and pastel stucco houses with red tile rooftops set into the terraced hillside among tall cypress and towering palms, and bright red bougainvillea spilling over walls—my own private Tuscany.

It seemed all of us had much to celebrate. Copies of the Greek edition of my book, *The Brazilian Healer with the Kitchen Knife*, had just arrived in the mail, bringing the number of translations to seven. Masha was soon to be off to the Sea of Japan to begin shooting her underwater film documentary. Sebastian, Masha's man and a wonderful cellist, would be starting work on a new opera. Terry and Jan were planning their trip to Paris. Alex was just back from Brazil with a wonderful little painting of a Candomblé ceremony (the very ceremony I was writing about in my novel). Julie Adams was newly in love with Andrew, a man she'd known 30 years before and who had just turned up in her life again. I would soon be going back to Brazil to continue research on the book. The first half of the decade had been good to all of us; the second half promised to be even better.

My books have been good to me. They have taken me to meet spiritual leaders of Native American tribes across the United States and Canada; to Dharamsala, India to meet with one of the greatest beings of our time, His Holiness the Dalai Lama; and, to healers in Brazil who make the blind see, the crippled walk, and who make tumors disappear with nothing more than an ordinary kitchen knife.

In northern India I climbed rugged mountains to interview lamas in their ancient monasteries. One September a few years ago on my birthday, Betty Fussell, author and world traveler, joined me in Ladakh (she in her safari hat); and we climbed 14,000 feet to a tiny remote eleventh-century village to meet the oracle of Wanla (who took a liking to Betty's hat and wanted to be photographed in it). Afterward, we scrambled back down the mountain, slipping and sliding and grabbing at bush branches, to meet the crone who lived in a cave-like dwelling at the bottom.

Almost crawling, we made our way into the crone's cave. She was sitting, knees drawn up on the bare earthen floor. She talked to us about her life of prayer. Each night before she goes to sleep, she said, she prostrates to the Buddha and prays that all her wrong actions from the past be pardoned. As we were leaving, she asked us whether we were happy. She wondered whether all our fine clothes and furniture and riches kept us too busy to find time for prayer. "But I'm just an old lady," she said. "I don't know about such things."

Oh, she knew all right. I didn't know it then, but her musings about us would become an important aspect of the spiritual path that lay before me, the beginnings of the lessons my books would teach me—provided of course I was willing to set aside all my fine clothes and furniture and riches that kept me so busy.

A few days later as I walked the narrow streets of Dharamsala with tattered and sun-bleached prayer flags fluttering from every doorway and window, I became aware of a constant hum, a low-pitched rumble that seemed to emanate from deep inside the earth. The sound rose through the soles of my feet, vibrating in me and around me, then was carried on the wind to the jagged mountain peaks, where it dissolved into pure light.

I did not discover the source of that sound until the day I walked down the hill to the Dalai Lama's residence just past the monastery. As I drew closer, the hum grew louder and louder. In a huge outdoor hall, several hundred Tibetan monks, young and old, sat cross-legged in their saffron robes chanting, their voices like the ocean's roar. Transfixed, I stopped.

The little monks, no bigger than kindergartners, sat in the last row shooting spitballs at the monks in the row in front of them who never once broke their concentration. The chant master soon came up behind the little ones and swatted them with a stick. I smiled. Anyone could see that they were spiritual spitballs.

One of the rimpoches—Tibetan for precious one, an honorific given to a master teacher—explained to me that the chants, which are the Buddha's teachings, do indeed reach into the earth and into the trees, rocks and streams, where gods and spirits live. Even to the hawks that circle overhead, all sentient beings are benefited and blessed by the sacred sounds.

The sounds are a part of me, too; I carry them still. I can hear them in my meditations and when I take my walks in the hill behind my apartment building. Gods and spirits live there as well.

· · · · · · · · · · · ·

Life changes in a flash—mid-breath, mid-song. One minute I am unloading the dishwasher, hand-drying wine glasses and dust-busting crumbs from underneath the coffee table. In the next I am doubled over by a sharp pain in my right side. After a few minutes it goes away. A stitch, a pulled muscle, I think; but, that night, as I get into bed I notice it again. I decide it must be a bladder infection. I've had them in the past; the pain is familiar. I'll call my doctor in the morning.

That night I dream of the *Mimosa Pudica*, the strange Brazilian plant also known as the Sensitive Plant. I had seen one in Rio in the Jardin Botannical and found it scary—a small, pretty tropical shrub with fernlike leaves that quickly fold together when the plant is touched, recoiling. When the hand is withdrawn, the leaves unfold and the plant assumes its original form. I wake up with my heart pounding. That morning I notice blood in my urine.

My doctor is out of town. I'm going for lunch in Malibu at Carol Moss's house in the Colony. When I call to confirm our date, she reminds me about the small Urgent Care Clinic nearby. I decide to stop there on the way to Malibu to get a prescription for antibiotics. A pleasant young doctor examines a urine specimen and informs me I do have a bladder infection. I get the prescription filled at the corner drugstore.

Lunch at Carol's is always wonderful; she's a magnet. Dagmo-la Sakya, a Tibetan princess, is in town to give her Green Tara teachings and initiations. Hers was the first Tibetan family to settle in the States after the Chinese invasion; and she and her husband, H.H. Dagchen Rimpoche, founded a monastery in Seattle. I met and spent time with them when I was writing The Book of Tibetan Elders, and I attended their meditations. My interviews with Damog-la were really teachings, though I didn't understand that at the time. When she spoke of the sacred preciousness of motherhood, she asked me about my own mother. Reading the expression on my face and downcast eyes, she begged me to find that preciousness before it was too late. "I'll try," I said. "No, not try," she answered sternly. Since then she's written her own book, *Princess in the Land of Snows.*

During lunch at Carol's, Damog-la tells a story about when she first came to America. She had remarked to a woman she'd just met how beautifully old she looked. The poor woman was shocked. "I really don't understand Western society's fear of age," Damog-la says to us. "In Tibetan society, when you meet somebody for the first time, you ask their name then you ask their age." An *L.A. Times* journalist sitting next to her laughs and suggests she might not want to try that in Los Angeles. Another journalist, a TV anchor from Slovenia, agrees that ageism has taken hold in her country, too.

"Everybody wants to live a long life," Damog-la says. "But they don't want to grow old."

We all smile in recognition of this truth.

I am so involved in conversation that I almost forget to take the antibiotic.

· · · · · · · · · · · · ·

The next morning, Tuesday, I wake at five and discover more blood—lots of it. My doctor's back. Not satisfied with the diagnosis I was given at the Urgent Care Clinic, he sends me to an urologist. After a series of tests, he tells me another, slightly more invasive test is needed, a cystoscopy. Whoa. Whoa! Wait a minute, hold on there. What're we talking about here? We're not talking spiritual spitballs. We're talking about a test serious enough to require a general anesthetic so that a miniscule camera at the end of a long snake-like tube can be inserted through the urethra into the bladder and kidney. No. No! I want to refuse. I'm about to refuse, but I stop. On the other hand, that's not spiritual blood pouring out of me, is it?

I go through with it, and a new diagnosis comes back: I do not have a urinary tract infection. What I do have is a rare, fast-growing, high-grade, highly aggressive cancer.

This is the way it all changes: not with a bang, not with a whimper. It changes with a phone call from a very nice man, a doctor, who uses his first name and says he is very sorry. I stand at the window gazing out over the hills. The world has gone black and white, a film noir. The morning moon has dropped behind the Griffith Observatory, and the day is beginning. Sounds from the street—cars and buses and horns—are fuzzy, distorted, like a defective sound track. I notice with little more than passing interest that I have no tears.

I try to take stock. I am divorced and my children are married with children of their own. I have a wide circle of friends and a handful of close friends. It is my work that makes living alone okay, necessary even. Writing is a fine torment, an exquisite mad passion, and the only thing I know that is never a waste of time. Even when I'm writing badly, especially when I'm writing badly, then I have to learn my craft all over again.

My routine is to write in the morning. I am working on a novel, *Day of Yemanja,* set in Brazil against the backdrop of the esoteric religions and the magic and mysticism of that country. My protagonist is a painter, as obsessed with his art as I am with mine. His life, too, has hit a wall. He stands at the edge of the sea at midnight and stares at the moonlight on the sea, imagining himself walking out along that path of moonlight to wherever it leads. Behind him, a strange midnight ceremony is taking place, one that he will wander into.

I can hear the drumbeats of the ceremony as I write. I know that moonlight path. I can smell the sea. I too was drawn to the magic when I was in Brazil, especially the shamanistic rituals. I felt the power of them, felt them in every nerve of my body. If only I could will myself there now, before the doctors and the hospitals, before I have to walk the path that leads to the land of the ill.

By noon I break from my writing and have a bite of lunch, do errands, take a walk, check emails and make phone calls, pay bills. Sometimes I pick up my three-year-old grandson Billy at pre-kindergarten. We might go to Larchmont to the bookstore or to Jamba Juice for a mango smoothie. Then, I take Billy home to play games with his little brother, Daniel. In the evenings I see friends or stay home and read and do some editing on the morning's pages. My day has seldom included doctor appointments, except lately come to think of it, when I've had more than my share of achy, flu-like viruses.

This new information, this diagnosis, is going to become terribly time-consuming, I'm thinking. I don't define exactly what the *this* is exactly, the label that's been pinned on me. Just that I will probably be spending a lot of time in the waiting rooms of doctors' offices. I've got a book to finish, and I'm supposed to go to Brazil in February and to New York in March. This is most definitely not a good time.

I must take stock. First the children, there are six of them, including stepchildren and their children who are all scattered across the country. Except for middle son Billy, father of little Billy, who will, I'm afraid, wind up bearing the brunt of all this, because he lives nearby. In other, older cultures, aging, death and dying are part of the natural order of things. Not in ours. In our culture, aging, death and dying are a curse, certainly not to be mentioned in passing, as Damog-la did to the shocked woman in the grocery store. In our culture women do not want to be complimented on their beautiful older age.

I know Billy will handle this nobly. It's me I'm worried about. I had come to believe that all illnesses are rooted in one's spiritual and emotional ill health and that maybe the humming vibrations of Dharamsala were still a part of me and that I was somehow protected. I had learned from healers and shamans that everything, *everything* is energy and that more highly evolved a person, the higher the frequency. Did I assume that from years of exposure to these highly evolved energies and absorbing the teachings my frequency had been raised and my spiritual acumen automatically deepened? Was I mistaken? Or is cancer a disease that is outside the realm of spirituality?

There are practical considerations, too. I'm not sure how well I can handle the threat of losing my independence even for a while. (It *will* only be for a while, won't it?) Billy is a busy and successful film editor and director with a wife and two toddlers; this could turn out to be—I swallow hard—I could wind up being—dare I say it?—a considerable burden. I know I must bring my trepidations out in the open, but I'm not sure how. And what about finances, as I may not be so productive for a while. My nest-egg could all too soon disappear down a very deep hole.

No question, this Bad Thing is going to be hard on us all.

In Brazil I was warned of some hostile force that was making its way to me from a man I met at the Spiritist Center, a healing and educational hub outside of Rio where I was doing research for the novel. At the time I did not understand the meaning of what he said. Bebeto, my augurer, is himself a healer, as well as a documentary filmmaker, who volunteers as a translator for the other healers at the Center whenever he can.

"You must gather your resources," he said. "An extreme change is coming to your life, a hostile force that will cause you to lose your way for a while. When you find it again, your life will be *"transportada."* We had exchanged phone numbers, as he planned to be in Los Angeles working on a project for a few months.

When I got back to the hotel, I looked up the word in my pocket-size dictionary. "Transported" was the definition. I still couldn't figure out what he meant. I think of this encounter now in the light of the diagnosis, "the hostile force," I was just hit with and wonder: Transported, as in passing from this life to the spirit world?

I think of the words of Pete Catches, holy man of the Lakota Sioux: "We do not inherit the world from our ancestors; we borrow it from our children."

I will have to tread very carefully. As much as I will need the children's love and support, I must remember that this journey is mine not theirs.

Bill Johnson brought to our marriage his three daughters, Wendy, Sally and Debbie, ages 10, 8 and 4. I brought my two-year-old son, Mark. Together we had two more sons, Billy and Anthony. After that we stuck to puppies.

When I met Bill, he was a Broadway producer; I was a young actress. I auditioned for a play he was co-producing with his brother-in-law, David Wayne, who was also starring in the production. The reading took place in a darkened theater, I remember; I had to read with the bored, drowsy stage manager, who could barely stay awake to feed me the damn lines.

My irritation informed my reading, which was totally inappropriate for the sweet ingénue character I was auditioning to play. From somewhere behind the stage-lights, a voice asked me to start again. Peering into the dark, I asked, "Start from where?" "The top," the voice answered, a bit impatiently. My reading got no better, and the voice in the dark thanked me and called for the next actress.

Not surprisingly, I did not get the part. Some months later, I was in a soap opera. I became friends with Susan Slade, the production assistant, who had once worked for Bill. She invited him to come watch the taping of the show from the control booth at CBS. When the camera zoomed in for my close-up, Bill turned to Susan and said, "That one. Terrible actress. That's the girl I'm going to marry."

One night many years later at dinner in a favorite restaurant over New Zealand mussels in a sauce of white wine and shallots, Bill looked at me with dark serious eyes and said, "I never want to be a burden on the children." It was at the very beginning of his illness.

I said, "No, nor do I. Let's make a pact. Let's only be a 'burden' to each other."

"No," said Bill, who was more than a decade older than I, "Not on you, either."

He kept his word.

Amid the cold and deep

snows of midwinter,

the wolf packs howled hungrily

outside Indian villages.

The people kept the fires going

and sang their songs until they

could no longer hear the

sound of the wolves.

Sioux

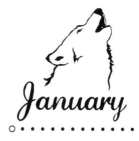

January

THE MOON OF THE TERRIBLE

On a table in the living room is a collection of carved turtles that I picked up during my travels through Indian country for *The Book of Elders: Life Stories & Wisdom of Great American Indians*, miniatures fashioned from stone, bronze, pewter and other materials. I pick up a silver one that I bought at a trading post near the Pine Ridge Indian Reservation in South Dakota and turn it over in my hand, remembering. The owner of the store had explained that the turtle represents Earth.

"See, there are 13 large scales on Old Turtle's back, one for each month of the year," he said.

When I looked at him quizzically, he explained, "Lakota moons did not follow today's twelve-month calendar; the Lakota moons follow each season. Spring, summer and fall each have three moons, while winter has four."

He pointed to the small scales that surround the large ones. "These 28 small scales represent each day in a lunar month. All together, they hold the key to the mysteries of the moon." Then he added, "For those who know how to look." The way the ancients kept track of the seasons was to give names to each of the full moons: January is the Moon of the Terrible; February, the Ice Moon; March, the Crow Moon; April, the Moon of the Awakening; May, the Moon When the Ponies Shed Their Shaggy Hair; June, the Spider Moon; July, the Moon of the Sacred Sundance; August, the Moon of the Joyful; September, the Moon of Change; October, the Hunter's Moon; November, the Thanking Moon; and December is the Turning Moon.

"But you said there were thirteen scales," I said. "What is the thirteenth?"

"Ah that," he said with a secret smile, "That moon is for the time of dreaming, of magic: it is the sacred time."

. . . .

As the months passed during my year of living tremulously, there were moons that watched as I walked purposefully, head erect, spine straight, but there were also times when the moon's face—the goddess whose light ruled the night—was turned away from me. Those nights were silent and dark, and I staggered and stumbled. Once or twice, when no one was around to see, I even melted into a puddle of grief. But still no tears. Never tears.

. . . .

In this Moon of the Terrible, I am in the land of hospital waiting rooms. I am assigned a patient number and a new ID by an admittance person with alarmingly long blood-red nails. She somehow manages to type my entire medical history, along with a good deal of my personal story, into a computer—marriages, divorces, pregnancies, children, smoking, drinking, drugs. Do I wear a seat belt while driving? *What???* Then come the doctors, the ones the Hopi call the White Coats.

Another receptionist leads me down a long hall to a row of offices past framed prints of sunsets in the desert, wild horses galloping across the prairie, wildflowers on a mountainside, and a sailboat in a calm sea. She ushers me into the end corner office with its blinds closed against the noonday sun, blocking out a living tableau. The doctor, an oncologist, does not rise to greet me but looks up from the files on his desk and mumbles his name and nods in the direction of the chair opposite him. "I see here that you've been diagnosed with a high grade…" he mumbles, looking in my general direction. I did not get the rest of the sentence.

"Sorry?" I ask, leaning forward.

"Incurable…controllable," are the words I get; but, since he doesn't look at me—he is looking straight ahead now at his computer screen—I don't get which of those words applies to me.

"Start protocol…chemotherapy…two weeks on, two off… right away…see Mrs.…(?) to set up appointments…explain everything…" The phone on his desk rings. "Excuse me," he says and turning his back to me, he picks it up.

I stand. "Excuse me," I say and open the door to leave.

He glances up. "Next week," he says, I think to me.

I run past the flaming sunset, the galloping horses, the wild-flowers, and the sailboat to the bank of elevators. Looking back as if to make sure no one is chasing me, I get in and lean against the handrail for support.

At my next appointment with my own doctor, Keith Agre, he hugs me and misty-eyed, assures me that I can beat this. He even tells me how: with my mind. Now Keith Agre is not a power-of-positive-thinking kind of guy. He's a pragmatist who understands me and how fiercely determined I am. He's been my doctor ever since I moved to L.A. ten years before, and we have an easy, warm relationship. We discovered we grew up less than a mile apart outside Philadelphia and share a love of music, an interest in politics which we sometimes agree on. Where we part ways, not surprisingly, is anything, *anything* about alternative medicine, which includes vitamins and supplements, nutrition and, of course, energy healing.

Billy is with me. In terms we can understand, Keith carefully explains the type of cancer I have and how it can be treated. Billy takes notes. I have the feeling he is also keeping an eye on me to make sure I don't bolt for the door and run off to one of my shamans to drink potions made from the eyeballs of boiled rattlesnakes; or, to Brazil to one of the healers in my book, which is what part of me wants to do. The part of me that longs for another kind of healing, the kind of healing that I know from my research, as well as my experience, is out there. Although Keith is an excellent clinician and sensitive to my needs, it would be useless to try to discuss the deeper spiritual matters that are going through my mind, energy healing, for instance, that might get to the root of the disease and prevent its spread. I have seen the evidence; this would be the time to go and apply it to myself.

Somehow I don't, though. It's out of my hands now. I have entered the Land of Cancer, governed by White Coats, through a passageway where I am blindfolded, spun round and round, and pointed in one direction or another. If there is a door leading out, at this moment I cannot see it.

Billy and I share many of the same sensibilities with the exception of anything remotely related to the world of healers. The very mention of this world will drive him right out of his linear, strong-minded and quite opinionated head. When my book on healers came out a couple of years before, he made no bones about hating the subject matter (though he was careful to preface his remarks by saying he thought the book was well written).

This middle son of mine, with his father's darkly serious eyes, has grown to be my protector. Not just because he is the one who lives in L.A., but because it has always been his role in the family. I'm guessing he feels what I need protecting from is myself.

They fly in: Mark, the eldest, from New Hampshire; Anthony, the youngest, from New Mexico; Sally from Florida; Wendy from northern California. Debbie, who lives in New York with her two boys, is in the middle of a nasty divorce; she writes thoughtful, loving notes. We are a tight tribe, we Johnsons—do not mess with us. We close ranks and guard each other fiercely. Their love takes my breath away.

Sally is in town to give an acting workshop with Dee Wallace. She has set aside extra days to go with me to medical appointments. Sunday, Billy and his wife HJ make us one of their elaborate brunches of poached eggs, bacon (why not?), English muffins, fresh fruit and steaming cappuccinos.

Billy and Sally are laughing, swapping stories about their father's sometimes riotously quirky behavior (getting on an airplane in his sheepskin bedroom slippers or how in a car he would reach over and grab the steering wheel—his way of giving directions). HJ and I are discussing the pros and cons of having two kids practically in one litter (their boys are 14 months apart) or having them as I did, five years apart.

Afterward, Sally and I go outside and sit on the hammock, little boys crawling all over us. When they run off, Sally puts her head on my shoulder and cries. I feel such love for them; they are my reason.

Moments like these make me think this moon doesn't seem all that terrible, until toward the end of it, on the 27th day. I am in Keith Agre's office for a routine appointment. I am sitting on the examining table talking to Billy, who sits with his notebook in the chair facing me. Keith behind me makes his examination: listening to my heart, tapping my back to check the lungs. Then he feels around my neck, stopping when he comes to the area of my right collarbone.

"What's this?" he asks.

I put my hand there. I don't feel anything. Maybe a tiny bump.

"I think we need to have this biopsied," he says.

I look across at Billy, then I turn to Keith and frown disapprovingly, as though he has just stepped out of line. I had agreed to something bad in my kidney, but that's all I signed on for. Do not go poking around looking for more trouble.

I probably didn't say any of this.

On the way home, Keith calls me on the cell phone. "They have a bed for you at Cedars. Tomorrow."

"Tomorrow?"

"Get there at six."

"Six in the morning?"

"Right," he says and rings off.

"I don't have any nice nightgowns," I turn and say to Billy.

Billy pretends this is a perfectly reasonable response.

Sally and I head for Nordstrom's at the Grove. We pass the chocolate counter just inside the entrance, ignoring the delicious aroma, and make our way through clouds of perfume from the cosmetic counters to the shoe department. There's a sale going on, and the place is swarming with Hollywood girls in tight minis and six-inch heels, their hair the colors of anything but hair. I watch them as they pull jewel-encrusted cell phones out of designer bags, a pack of cigarettes toppling to the floor, and wonder what lies ahead for them. *Forever* is what I suspect they would say.

It is what I would have said.

The little nodule in my neck turns out to be malignant, a miniscule expeditionary force (a mass of one billion cancer cells cannot be detected by even the most advanced medical equipment) that escaped the terrorist camp in my kidney and sneaked past the 20 trillion immune cells that were supposed to be keeping watch. Were they unarmed? Hadn't they had their broccoli that day? It made its way to the right supraclavicular lymph node inside the collar bone to set up a new camp. The new diagnosis was metastatic Transitional Cell Cancer, (TCC). This puts me at Stage IV.

"Is there a Stage V?" I ask.

"No," the surgeon answers.

"I see."

I look over at Billy and Sally. They are standing quite still, their faces pale.

"Well then," I say. "We better fix it."

Both the surgeon and the oncologist tell me that this type of high-grade TCC travels fast to the lungs, liver or bone, therefore a new strategy is devised. They will systematically blast the cancer with medical weapons of mass destruction, top-of-the-line chemo. When I am sufficiently recovered from the chemo, remove the kidney.

This last part I did not hear. My mind had come to a halt at the mention of chemo. Every healer, shaman and medicine man I had ever known said the same thing: Once a person has had chemo, the body is too poisoned to receive healing.

I look at the faces of my children. Billy's eyes are fixed on me as if he is reading my thoughts.

When I was diagnosed with breast cancer 15 years ago, I said I was not going to have chemo. Bill and Billy ganged up on me, and I caved. I can blame that decision on them, or I can own up to my own lack of courage to follow the dictates of my beliefs. It's a runaway train, this cancer diagnosis, careening down a perilously steep hill. No way to slam on the brakes and give myself time to think. I'm well into the Land of Cancer now.

Moments later, Anthony comes rushing into the hospital room and, sobbing, throws himself onto the bed. We have a code, he and I. Bill died wearing his favorite shirt, an orange fleece pullover which we kept on him during the days and nights we sat vigil at the funeral chapel.

"Don't you go chasing the orange shirt, Mama," Anthony warns. "Promise me."

He says it again now. "Promise."

"I promise," I whisper.

· · · · · · · · · · · ·

At night, after everyone has gone and I am alone in the hospital room, which is dark now except for the ghastly yellow rectangle of light under the door, I do not take the pain pill or the sleeping pill. I am in no hurry for tomorrow. Instead, I reach for my notebook and turn on the bedside lamp. I prefer to spend these precious hours in my other world. Writing has always been my doorway into another world, one that I fashion out of my dreams. I walk easier there. I understand the people I find there. They make far more sense than the crazy irrational ones that walk around this ordinary world.

A nurse comes into the room and switches on the harsh, overhead light so suddenly that I raise my arms to shield my eyes. She takes my temperature, checks my blood pressure and asks if I need anything. I shake my head no. She insists that I take my pill and stands over me while I wash it down with water. I am on this side of the looking glass now, a captive in the Land of Cancer during the Moon of the Terrible. I drift into a dark, dreamless sleep to the sound of the wolves howling outside the door.

As a new moon arrived,

the Lakota people noticed a great

change. Trees on the Great

Plains popped and burst as their

branches became laden with winter

snow and ice. The people huddled

around the fire listening to the

stories the Elders told.

Lakota Sioux

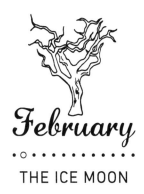

February

THE ICE MOON

January 20, 2006

Hi Everyone,

I apologize for the mass email. I've spoken to all of you at least once since the original report on Jan. 13, and now that more info is in I thought it easiest to just get everyone on the same page.

Here's the update: After weeks of waiting, punctuated by a variety of tests and scans, we've arrived at a diagnosis of Sandy's cancer and have been given a suggested course of treatment.

Basically, she's got a high-grade cancer which has metastasized to other areas of her body from the original site in her kidney. This type of cancer (a relatively uncommon form of kidney cancer) has no known cure, and the goal is to control it through chemotherapy. The treatments are not expected to bring on hair loss or extreme nausea.

The plan to remove her kidney was abandoned when the metastases were discovered; the diseased kidney is still functioning well and will be needed to remove the byproducts of the chemotherapy. Also she'll be stronger if she hasn't just had an organ removed.

The pain is being controlled to some extent by Vicodin, which

*makes her a bit loopy at times, so she uses it judiciously. Sitting upright
for extended periods causes her a lot of discomfort (it's kind of like a bad
case of sciatica), so don't invite her to a Wagner opera or a long dinner
until the pain begins to subside, hopefully soon.*

*She looks great, by the way, and she is her usual loving wonderful
self through all of this.*

*Though she feels a little overwhelmed right now, my sense is that
your calls and even visits/invitations will be most welcome in the
coming days and weeks.*

*We are going to be actively seeking other opinions before the
proposed chemo starts on Thursday. If your first cousin just got the
Nobel for nephro-oncology, now's the time to pick up the phone. On
the other hand, if you have a healer in Sedona you want her to meet,
please be reminded: she wrote the book—literally—on faith/alterna-
tive healers, and as of this time she has chosen not to contact any of the
many interesting individuals depicted therein.*

Thank you for all of your calls and support.

Billy

Huddled in winter under the February moon, chilly and
damp even in Southern California, the family assembles around
me as chemo treatments begin. Like the snow-laden branches of
the trees on the Great Plains, my bones have turned to ice. I ask
the doctors whether it's the disease that's making me so cold or
the chemo. The oncologist says it's the disease, Keith Agre says it's
the chemo. I think the cause of my deep chill is fear of both the
disease and the cure. I pile on sweaters as everyone else peels off
theirs, and we tighten the circle against the approaching storm.

Each child comes offering a story, a memory, fresh baked, newly observed, or retrieved from the treasure trove of our shared past. "Remember the time Anthony tried to ride his bike off the roof of the garage?" Or, "What was the name of that girlfriend of Mark's who gave him pot?"

We dig into boxes of photographs and letters that have survived my countless moves: New York, Santa Fe, Maryland for a teaching stint at Washington College, Palm Beach for a year to be near my 92-year-old mother, then back to Santa Fe, and finally, here to L.A. Those sagging and tattered boxes of photographs and letters are always with me; they are my proof.

We laugh as we read them aloud to each other. Wendy, spending a semester on a kibbutz in Israel, wrote "My job here is to get up at five each morning and wash chicken shit off all the eggs. A job strictly reserved for Christian girls." She wanted to stay in Israel and get a job teaching, but the Israeli government wouldn't issue her a license unless she agreed to convert to Judaism. "...And I thought Israel was supposed to be a new land of freedom!" Thoughtful, quiet Wendy became head gardener and a lay teacher at Green Gulch Zen Center in northern California and is about to publish her first book, *Gardening at the Dragon's Gate*. She reads a passage to me in which she quotes a saying of the Buddha, one that applies to me in my life as it is in this moment: "The one who sits down in the middle of his life and looks with attention, calm and resolute, has a chance to untangle the tangle and to relieve suffering."

Sally, blond, outgoing, middle step-daughter, became an actress and then an acting teacher with her own studio in New

York. As we talk about our acting days, memories come flooding in. There was the filming of "Ash Wednesday" on location in Cortina, a ski resort in northern Italy with Elizabeth Taylor, Henry Fonda and the German actor Helmut Berger (I played his girlfriend, and in one scene I had to slap him across the face. It took several takes to get the scene right, so I had raw filet mignons sent up to his room that night). Henry and I went trudging through the snow to shop for gifts, I remember. Richard Burton visited the set, and he and Elizabeth fought like mad, forever reprising their roles as George and Martha, it seemed.

Mark, with his over-the-top IQ, had become a computer whiz and environmentalist. On a visit to L.A. to speak at the Audubon Society, Mark plays handyman around my apartment, keeping my computer running so that I can continue to write of the dark happenings in Brazil.

Billy, who after seeing "Those Magnificent Men in their Flying Machines" and "Oliver" at least a dozen times at age nine, decided that he would become a filmmaker and did.

Anthony skied through prep school, partied through college, and wound up a successful commercial realtor. Finally, Debbie, who always loved clothes, became a true Dress-up Princess, working as a couturier in her own atelier on Manhattan's Upper East Side.

They are smart, loving and forthright people, endlessly interesting, each with his or her own brand of wit; they are my favorite people on earth. Watching them grow as their characters unfolded and their lives took shape was like reading a good book; I can't wait to turn the page and see what happens in the next chapter. And their children—who will they turn out to be? I wonder whether in the spirit world I'll be able to hang around and watch them. Are spirits subject to the laws of gravity, or do they just go drifting off into orbit and become a part of the Earth's halo of space junk? Will I weep missing them so?

I come across a poem I had copied; I think after I had been diagnosed with breast cancer. Strange, but I don't remember having the feelings at the time that would resonate so strongly with this poem written by South American poet, Cesar Vallejo.

> *I will die in Paris, on a rainy day,*
> *on some day I can already remember.*
> *I will die in Paris—and I don't step aside—*
> *perhaps on a Thursday, as today is Thursday, in*
> *autumn.*
> *It will be a Thursday, because today, Thursday,*
> *setting down these lines, I have put my upper arm*
> *bones on wrong, and never so much as today have I*
> *found myself with all the road ahead of me, alone.*

And here I am again—not alone, though, except in the sense that we are all alone.

My determination to live blinds me, and the evidence I am presented with paralyzes. This particular cancer is high-grade, fast-growing, I'm told, one that with chemo might be controlled for a few (three? five?) years, depending on how I respond to treatment. It is not curable. This is gospel according to the White Coats. The certainty of that statement blots out for the moment all I once thought I knew. I have seen with my own eyes the spontaneous, miraculous healings in Brazil and India and on Indian reservations across this country, which now suddenly seem a far-off dream. There are also the reports of people who with nothing more than prayer and meditation were able to heal themselves without any medical intervention.

It is because belief has momentarily abandoned me that I sit here on this fake leather recliner while poisons flood my body, poisons, I'm told, that will kill many of the billions of cancer cells that have taken root in me and will also destroy my immune system. But only for a while, they assure me.

What if this cancer is the result of the chemo I had 15 years earlier, when I had a bout with breast cancer? When I ask the oncologist, I'm told no, this is not the same type of cancer cell. Wait a minute. It's still cancer, isn't it? It's still cells that have gone haywire, right? What is it in my body that permits cells to go haywire? My immune system, right? What if I were one of those people able to strengthen my own immune system sufficiently for my body to shake off the cancer cells?

I had posed these questions to Keith Agre before beginning treatment. He listened and shook his head sadly and said he wishes that were so. "Believe me, if that were possible, we'd know about it." He explained the course that this disease of mine would take without medical intervention. The cancer would go to the liver, the bones, the brain. He delivered this verdict firmly, matter-of-factly.

In other words, *Do what we tell you to do and you might live.*

I am not after all, Native American or Tibetan or for that matter a Brazilian Spiritist. I am a Westerner living in this time. Much as I may choose to believe in other more ancient, more spiritual values, Western conventional medicine is what I have been programmed to believe in.

Nights when I am alone in the blackest of hours, the demons' hours, they come. I lie very still, barely able to breathe. My heart banging against my chest. I know these demons; I remember them well from childhood. Tree monsters, I used to call them, gnarled and dwarfed dryads, creatures of the nighttime forest come to take me away. I would scream the household awake then, until someone (I preferred my father, he listened better than my mother) came to turn on lights and stay with me until I was sure the monsters had retreated. My father, with his tender eyes so full of compassion is not here to calm and comfort me; he passed away long ago. Instead, bravely I reach for the bedside light, squeezing my eyes shut until I think the demons have gone. Wide awake then, I escape into the parallel world that unfolds in the spiral notebook beside my bed. I'd been working on my character Sara's conversation with the medium, also called a shaman (the one I/she met when she visited the Spiritist Center and the one she went to while her husband Peter sealed himself off in the hotel room painting.)

"There is no death," the shaman explained. "Existence does not end with the passing of the physical body. Nor does the spirit go to some far distant place. Spirits are right here beside us, guiding and healing and teaching us. Above all, loving us. Unconditionally, without judgment."

Helping us heal as well? Do I dare believe I can be healed by blending conventional *and* alternative medicine? More importantly, how essential is my belief that I can be healed? If it isn't strong enough, how do I begin to strengthen my beliefs that I may overcome my fear? Not of death, it is not death I fear; it is dying.

That must have been what Bill feared too: not the pain, but the loss of control, the loss of self, and the loss of every last shred of power over one's own life or over one's death for that matter. We know the scene; it's cliché. The patient lies in the hospital bed, tubes coming out of everywhere hooked up to machines. Not dead, but no longer in the world of the living. A holding cell. Poked and prodded by strangers. Doctors looking up from their clipboards, peering, but not really seeing; speaking, but not really talking, guarding against their own sense of futility. Children standing around the bed, trying hard to be brave and comforting; friends trying hard to hide their own fears.

I find I am drawn to books about dying, both fiction and non-fiction. Stories told by people in the spirit world, and books and movies about people dying nobly. I rent the DVD of the film, *Evening*, with Vanessa Redgrave in which she is a woman dying beautifully, elegantly at home in her own bed, a nurse in attendance, her two daughters near. She relives scenes from her life, floating in and out of the present, seamlessly drifting toward death. I run the film again and study Redgrave's performance. When it is my time that is how I should like to leave this world, even though I know a spiritually enlightened person should be able to accept whatever life presents, even a not-so-pretty hospital kind of end.

An astrologer once offered to tell me the time of my death. It was in India when I was researching my book on Tibetan elders. In Dharamsala, the Tibetan Institute of Medicine and Astrology is near the Dalai Lama's residence. Astrology plays an important role in all aspects of Tibetan life, from government to marriage and to matters of health. In fact medical students are required to study astrology. His Holiness suggested I visit the Institute and ask Jampa Kalsang to do my chart. No book on Tibetan culture would be complete without including the subject of astrology. Most Tibetans wish to know the time of death, so that they can prepare for a good rebirth; I made it clear at the outset that I did not wish to know the time of mine. A person's life span can be calculated, he explains, but it can also be shortened by earthquake, war or terminal illness, unless one has the karmic potential to survive. The Tibetan word for star is karma; one's karma is written in the stars. I learned that I have a windy and phlegmatic nature, that I promote frequent changes of feeling and residence, that I love to meet new people and exchange ideas, that my weakness could be impatience, and that my life could "end up with poison, so always be aware." Jampa Kalsang did not, as requested, give me the date of my death, but the chart does come to an abrupt end right around the age of 70. I leave Jampa Kalsang wondering if the Tibetan stars really held a message for me. What was the poison they spoke of?

I ponder that as I climb the steps to the temple that houses ancient Buddha statues, wall hangings and deities, and find myself standing in front of the towering statue of Mahakali, the wrathful form of Tara. Fierce and grotesque, face and figure blue, she looks down at me with blood-red angry eyes. Also known as the warrior mother who fights against the forces of human imperfection, bondage and death, Mahakali is said to shed bitter tears for those who refuse to transcend their limitations of ignorance and darkness.

I think of my relationship with my mother and my inability to express to her my feelings of anger and hurt, letting them fester instead over the years, and wonder if that could be the poison Jampa Kalsang spoke of. Poison that would one day become the cancer that would threaten my life.

Later on during that same trip, while interviewing the Dalai Lama, I would ask him if it is possible to change one's karma, even though it is written in the stars. He assured me it was, with prayer, good deeds, and most of all, consciousness. Prayer and good deeds. I'm not sure I've done enough of either. Is it too late? I must re-read Pema Chödrön, a Tibetan nun who wrote, *Start Where You Are*. Our one duty to life is simply to live it, the great teachers say, to meet our karma straight on. So, it was karma then that I was born to a mother who was in some ways like Mahakali, except that her idea of imperfection was me not agreeing with her, not accepting the limitations that she tried to instill in me. Having a mind of my own, as she put it, is what inspired her wrath.

Consciousness is all, I decide. It is the light that dissolves fear. This lifelong quest of mine for consciousness, this, too, is my karma.

After the long winter when

Darkness threatened to last forever

and the snows never seemed to stop,

groups of crows stayed close

together to create their own source

of light and safety.

Cherokee

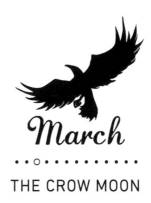

March

· · ○ · · · · · · · · · ·

THE CROW MOON

A device the size and shape of a watch battery is installed in my upper right arm just beneath the skin. It works like this. There's a small intake at one end which protrudes through the skin and at the opposite end is a very thin blue tube about 18 inches long that connects to the superior vena cava. The purpose of the device is to avoid repeated poking to draw blood for labs and for delivery of chemo and to prevent damage to the veins. I pretend it also doubles as a communications device enabling me to consult doctors in other galaxies (known in Brazil as Spirit Doctors) when I want a second opinion, especially when doctors on this planet talk to me about percentages and survival rates.

I do what my doctors had warned me not to do, my own research. Too scary, they said. A little knowledge is dangerous, they said, you'll scare yourself to death. Really? Well, if I'm going to die anyway, I prefer to die with eyes wide open (so to speak).

Like the crows of the March Moon in the Cherokee legend who lighted fires and covered their dwellings with layers of blankets, I will create my own source of light and safety with knowledge. I call Margery Nelson, who's been a friend ever since our days at the Lee Strasberg Studio. Margery and I did a scene from a J.D. Salinger short story, "Uncle Wiggly in Connecticut." I moved back to New York, but Margery remained in California and married Bill Link, who with his partner Dick Levinson created *Columbo, Murder She Wrote* and many more TV series and some wonderful theater plays too. Margery puts me in touch with Marcia Horn, a woman in Arizona who serves as president of International Cancer Advocacy Group, a cancer research foundation. Marcia is an invaluable source for translating doctor and lab reports into terms that a frightened patient can understand. Knowledge *is* empowering.

I spend days in the Los Feliz Library deep in research. I learn that the word cancer comes from the Greek physician Hippocrates, who used the word *karkinos* (crab) to describe the hard swellings and ulcerations he saw in the breast or protruding from the rectum or vagina. The finger-like spreading projections called to mind the shape of a crab.

Hippocrates believed that the body contained four humors (body fluids): blood, phlegm, yellow bile, and black bile. A balance of these fluids resulted in a state of health. Any excesses or deficiencies caused disease. An excess of black bile collecting in various body sites was thought to cause cancer. This theory of cancer remained the unchallenged standard for over 1300 years. Since the late Middle Ages, there has been a succession of theories, from fermenting and degenerating lymph fluid to trauma, parasites, environmental pollution, and more recently, viruses.

I reread Susan Sontag's *Illness as Metaphor* in which she

describes cancer as unromantic and cursed, unlike TB. Recall Marguerite in *La Dame aux Camelias* in a long white dress languishing on a silk pillowed chaise, or the more elegant heart murmur of Mrs. Dalloway. Sontag challenges the then popular notion that cancer is the result of repressed emotion over a trauma such as the loss of a parent, lover, spouse, or close friend.

This notion is even more popular now, especially among New Agers, who devour books that promote the belief that we cause our own cancer; and therefore, we can cure our own cancer. Popular psychologists like Lawrence LeShan have created a cancer personality type that is "dark, devoid of self, whose childhood is marked by feelings of isolation." Cancer is a modern day Black Plague, malignant, maligned.

What about all the many people who have suffered severe losses and traumas who do not have cancer? What about three-year-olds with leukemia? (Please don't talk to me about how we must suffer the consequences of deeds committed in past lives. As far as I'm concerned, that's as woolly-headed as the Twinkie Defense. I mean, I think I believe in reincarnation, I want to believe in reincarnation, but I'll have to get back to you on that.)

I learn that chemotherapy was born in the trenches of World War I, when mustard gas was used as a chemical warfare agent. Scientists discovered that mustard gas reduced the number of white blood cells, leading to the further discovery during World War II that the gas could also slow the rate of cancer cell division. Several patients with advanced lymphomas were given the drug by injection to avoid having to breathe the irritating gas, and their improvement, although temporary, was remarkable.

Later, in the Vietnam War, the United States used Agent Orange as part of its herbicidal warfare program to destroy crops and foliage. Researchers began to look for other substances that might have similar effects against cancer. They concluded that two naturally occurring substances, inositol and folic acid, inhibited the growth of breast cancer cells in mice, which led the scientists to wonder whether the drugs would be suitable for chemotherapy in humans.

The overall strategy is very like bombing a whole country in order to kill a handful of terrorists—a medical version of a scorched-earth policy. At that point, no one had yet found out how to perform a chemical version of the surgical airstrike, targeting the enemy and leaving the civilians alone. They have since, I recently read.

At my next appointment with the grim-faced oncologist, I force myself to ask the hard question. Billy is with me again, taking notes. The office is small and stark with no sign of life—not a photograph or print or even a plant. Next to the computer on his otherwise bare desk sits a stack of papers neatly arranged, edges straight, corners perfectly aligned. The chairs are hard, the backs at an uncomfortable ninety-degree angle, and they are armless. Blinds are drawn against the sunlight and it is cold. Shivering, I pull my sweater around me.

Even with chemo, he answers in a voice so low I have to ask him to repeat what it was he has just said, I have but a five to seven percent chance of survival past three-and-a-half years. I blink my eyes and peer at him. Has he consulted with Jampa Kalsang?

He takes my quizzical expression to mean I want more

information about numbers, which I don't. He mumbles something about the survival percentages doubling and then tripling. I don't exactly get what that timetable means, but I think it's something about a tiny percent of patients living to die of something else, although I do not understand at what point that is. No matter; I have to find a way to make myself part of that doubling and tripling and finally the tiny percentage. I dig my trench, put on my helmet and hunker down.

So, like the crows who gather together in the last days of winter, I do what I always do in an emergency: I give a dinner party. An act of defiance or an act of faith? Maybe a little of both. I invite my favorite people, friends who somehow make me feel safe. I wear something pretty. In the depths of my closet I come across a bright blue and green silk jacket that Alex found for me in one of her secret shops. It will go nicely with black silk pants and a black silk tank-top.

With the addition of a leaf I can fit ten at my table. We will grill a rack of lamb (friends gather round the barbeque, drinks in hand, or hang out in the kitchen to help), roast tiny potatoes and top them with crème fraiche and red caviar (a potato version of my johnny cakes), and steam sugar snap peas with butter and dill. Endive and butter lettuce salad with my house vinaigrette, sorbet and ginger cookies for dessert, and a wonderful Malbec from Argentina. No one has to ask what the extra chair at the end of the table is for. We all know it is for the 1,200 pound gorilla in a clown suit who is the evening's unspoken guest of honor.

The subject of puppies comes up. Someone asks when I will get a new puppy. Tashi Delek, my adored nine-year-old Maltese, died a year-and-a-half before. He was my book present to myself when *The Book of Tibetan Elders* was published. I named him for the Tibetan words that mean "blessings and good fortune," and he lived up to his name. I had sent the Dalai Lama a picture of Tashi Delek, because he had told me that after his beloved Tibetan Terrier died, he realized he could never have another dog. It went against the Buddhist principle of non-attachment. I later learned His Holiness had put Tashi's picture on a wall in his quarters in Dharamsala.

I hesitate to answer the question of when I will get another puppy. "That would require a very large leap of faith," I answer.

The table falls silent. The gorilla in the clown suit has just taken his seat.

Sebastian has brought his cello. After dinner he plays the prelude to Bach's Cello Suite in G Major, a hauntingly beautiful piece. Time and space cease to exist. I am in that other dimension that knows no illness, where there is no beginning and no end. The magic is here. It hasn't left me after all.

I look around the room at my friends, who are also swept up in the moment. Our eyes meet, gentle love unspoken but sweetly felt passes between us.

I must hang onto this moment, especially tomorrow when I walk through the halls of the White Coats. I must keep it safe in my pocket where I can reach in and touch it, rub my fingers over it, and take it out and press it against my cheek. It will be my talisman against the killing aspect of my Janus-faced healers, Agent Orange and mustard gas.

Long ago all the people were healthy. When they grew old a shining spirit-messenger carried them up a magic vine to the sky where they lived forever. One day a grandmother climbed up the forbidden vine in pursuit of her grandson. The Great Spirit punished the people by sending sickness and death. But He also blessed them with the gift of healing.

Ojibwa

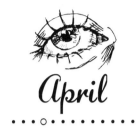

April

· · · · · ○ · · · · · · · · ·

THE MOON OF THE AWAKENING

The following day at my scheduled appointment with the oncologist, I try in vain to conjure the feeling of the night before, to hear again in my mind the strains of the music. It's no good. The magic's gone. No wonder. For one thing, it's too cold. They keep this place at meat-locker temperature. For another, it's the grim (reaper) oncologist who once again won't make eye contact, let alone speak clearly. It's obvious this is a man who doesn't believe, the sort of man who as a boy didn't clap for Tinker Bell. I was supposed to begin treatment on this day; I don't, there is no way I can heal in the hands of this man.

I must switch doctors. I leave the dour mumbler (who in all fairness has an excellent reputation) for an oncologist at USC's Norris Cancer Center, Dr. David Quinn. He's a great bear of a man, a cheerful Aussie who talks to Billy and me as if we were grown-ups. Keith Agre asked around among his colleagues and was told that Dr. Quinn was the best for my type of cancer. I ran his name past ICAG director Marcia Horn and she came up with raves. We don't meet in his office but in the examining room at Norris. I'm seated on the examination table, Billy in the upholstered armchair in the corner. Dr. Quinn leans his large frame, legs crossed, against the long nicely cluttered counter. He speaks in friendly, conversational tones, and seems genuinely interested that Billy is a film editor and director. They talk about the TV series Billy worked on, *House,* which Dr. Quinn promises to watch. He is also interested that I am a writer and had written about healers, among them an Australian aboriginal man. It's as if the last thing he wants to talk about is cancer. When we do finally get around to the subject at hand, he is optimistic. He asks if we have any questions. I think a moment and decide I don't. I will not get into the timetable-percentage numbers; I'll chart my own course, thanks anyway. "Then let's do this and get through it," Dr. Quinn says, "so you two can get back to your work."

. . . .

Billy and I are foodies. Ignoring the probability that chemo will destroy my taste buds, we are only half-joking when we assess which of our favorite eateries are nearby in deciding on a hospital. Norris is five minutes from Philippe's French Dip, and not far from a great dim sum restaurant, and Pho 87, a Vietnamese noodle place we love. Norris has free valet parking (you have to live in Los Angeles to know what a big deal that is). Norris and the Aussie win. Treatments will be two weeks on, two weeks off. Then come the PET/CT scans to see how I am responding. We celebrate our decision over Pho and strong Vietnamese coffee.

The huge chemo room is divided into curtained cubbies, each equipped with a recliner and a small TV. A pleasant Philippine nurse hooks me up to the IV and brings me a heated blanket.

61

I look up at the clear, innocent-looking liquid bulging in the plastic bag. See? Look, I tell myself, it's not orange at all, nor is it mustard-colored. And look, can't you see? It's going directly to the tumor cells, completely bypassing the healthy ones.

That is what I tell myself as I watch the drops fall one by one into the tube that leads to the delivery device in my upper arm that sends it drop by drop into my bloodstream. This is good medicine, medicine that will heal. I use Carl Simonton's Pac-Man image and visualize each drip turning into little yellow creatures that go straight to the enemy cells and gobble them up, one after the other. But then I get stuck in the scenario, trying to figure out where they go then. Do I excrete the yellow creatures stuffed with cancer cells and flush them down the toilet? Wait, don't they first have to go through the kidneys?

I decide instead to put on noise-cancelling earphones to drown out my neighbor's TV with Dr. Phil scolding some hapless husband who cheats on his wife. It gets me thinking how hard marriage was for me, thinking and remembering. I loved and respected Bill and liked him, too. We could sit up half the night talking about politics, books, movies, or reading. We so liked the same books that after one or the other of us had gotten half way through a book (paperback, of course), we'd cut it in half so we could both read it. Still, I couldn't seem to master marriage much beyond the ten-year marker.

I keep hearing the drips from the IV. Even through the earphones, I can hear each one, amplified it seems by the earphones. I take them off and listen instead to Oprah talking about the plight of fat people. I am about to turn it off when a woman comes on and begins to talk about her husband's decision to refuse continued treatment for a terminal, progressive illness, choosing instead to let the disease take its course, just keep him out of pain. He preferred to die at home with dignity, at a time of his choosing. The woman's daughter is angry at her for not insisting her father continue with treatment. I side with the father and the mother's support of that choice. I didn't, though, seven years ago when Bill made that same choice. I was devastated and enraged, and I later realized, betrayed.

We were already divorced (both of us having remarried and divorced again), when Bill fell ill with pseudo bulbar palsy, a debilitating disease similar to ALS, Lou Gehrig's disease. I was living in Santa Fe at the time; he was living an hour away in Albuquerque. We were seeing each other several times a week for dinner and sometimes a movie, and talking every day on the phone. We spent birthdays and holidays with whichever children were able to join us. We went Christmas shopping together, put up a tree and wrapped gifts and planned the holiday dinner. In our own way, we were a family again.

When Bill got sick, I divided my time between his house and mine, taking him to doctors' appointments and remaining at his side when he had to be hospitalized. "The divorce didn't take," he liked to explain to doctors and nurses.

Less than a year later, his illness had progressed to a point that was no longer tolerable to him. He chose December 7, 1998, Pearl Harbor Day. That had been his war (he was an Air Force lieutenant), and he did have a keen sense of history. Did he consciously choose to end his suffering on "the day that will live in infamy"? We don't know. We don't know for how long he planned it, either. When did he know no one would be in the house? I had left to go to Santa Fe, an hour away, for a lunch meeting. Billy was flying in from Los Angeles at three, and Anthony was picking him up at the airport. That gave Bill three hours, maybe four.

I was running late, and I needed to stop at my house in Santa Fe to pick up a few things: a change of clothes, perhaps; a book; the *New York Times* for Bill. The phone on the kitchen wall was ringing as I walked in the door. It was Billy's voice, choked, a sob. "It's Dad. He—took his life." I remember letting out a terrible howl—shock, horror, but most of all, rage. I sped along the interstate, blaming myself for leaving the house, blaming Bill for not talking it over with me (he had lost the ability to speak, but he was able to communicate by writing on a pad), for not giving me a chance to talk him out of it (maybe that was the point), and outrage that he had left it to our son to find him.

Over the coming days the word "dignity" was repeated over and over again, as well as the words "choice" and "control." He had to do it this way, Sally said, so as not to implicate any of us in his demise. Billy said Dad had chosen him to be the one to find him because he knew he could handle it. Like me, Wendy was furious. He had ducked out the back door, leaving without saying "I love you."

New Mexico had turned to ashes for me. I packed up and moved to L.A. Grief would have to wait.

· · · · · · · · · · · · ·

Seven years have passed. Now it's my turn to dance with mortality. I look up at the bag that hangs just over my head, dripping twentieth-century medicine drop by drop, medicine that may or may not heal for some yet-to-be-determined period of time. We, Bill and I, were always there for each other, in sickness and in health, even in divorce. We knew we could count on each other. I turn off the TV, letting Oprah settle the mother-daughter dispute over the father's decision to end his medical treatment, and close my eyes. Didn't you know that, Bill? I would have been there for you at your side right to the end. Just as I know you would be here for me now. I stop. A thought suddenly hits me: You took the option you chose away from me, Bill. Because no matter how gruesome this cancer I've been hit with might become, no matter how painful or debilitating, I am forced to live it out. Our children cannot have both parents leave this world by their own hand.

· · · · · · · · · · · · ·

It is Easter. I have now had five chemo treatments, and they are taking their toll. I limit my activities to one a day. I do not go grocery shopping on a day I have a doctor's appointment. If I meet a friend for lunch, I spend the rest of the day hanging out on the living room couch reading or, when I can, writing. I drift off to sleep so often that I have difficulty falling asleep at night and have to take an Ambien.

I'm also taking Vicodin from time to time to relieve the achiness caused by the chemo, and laxatives to combat the constipation caused by the Vicodin. That's on top of the anti-nausea pills, the occasional prescribed antibiotic when I run a fever, and three or four other drugs (including valium). Drug B to counter the effect of drug A, drug C to counter the effect of drug B, and on and on, until my body chemistry no longer recognizes itself. I can imagine my white cells thinking they're red cells, and red cells taking up arms against white cells. And my immune system collapsing under the confusion.

I pull myself together for Easter Sunday brunch at Billy's and HJ's. It is an exquisite day. Their large, gracious house with its sweeping lawns sits on the edge of a golf course, a perfect setting for them as superb hosts. Korean-born HJ is a high-powered executive who once worked as a caterer; Billy, himself a great cook, is a born nurturer. Friends and their little ones laugh and squeal and chase each other across the lawn. Little Billy wants me to watch him swing his golf club, and I am transported back in time to see his father at four or five hitting a golf ball on the driving range behind our house in East Hampton. Bill should be here to see this.

I can't help but notice my Emmy-Award-winning film editor son doing quite a lot of filming of me with his boys. I frown slightly in the direction of the camera. Capturing me for the archives because this might be my last Easter? But, Billy is smiling proudly, his face beaming with love. If that is what he's thinking, he's hiding it well. So am I, because the thought had crossed my drug-addled mind more than once.

The next night, Monday, before going to bed, I stand a moment at the living room window. This night I see the slender, intensely bright crescent moon: the ashy moon. This phrase I remember from my adored grandfather, who seemed to know everything about everything. It must have been an evening in early spring, perhaps April, since April and May are the months when the ashy moon is most pronounced, and June is when my grandfather died suddenly of a heart attack.

That April night, we were sitting outside, he and I, remarking on the sudden blossoming of the fragrant night jasmine, when he looked up at the sky and pointed to the crescent moon. "Look, the ashy moon." I had never seen it before or never noticed. But I have all the years of my life since. The slender crescent was bright, while the rest of the moon glowed dimly and, indeed, appeared the color of ash. My grandfather explained that ashy glow was caused by reflected sunlight from the earth or earthshine illuminating the moon's dark surface. "The story goes," my grandfather said, "that the New Moon is wishing that her lost love, the Old Moon, be in her arms one last time; Venus grants the wish." Then, seeing my adolescent eyes grow misty with the romance of it all, he quoted some lines from a poem by Emma Wilcox Wheeler, who I later learned much to my surprise, was a turn of the century mystic:

> *Swift thro' the vapors and the golden mist—*
> *The Full Moon's shadowy shape shone on the night,*
> *The New Moon reached out clasping arms and kissed*
> *Her phantom lover in the whole world's sight.*

On that night in early spring at the tender age of 14, I fell in love with the moon. For 20 years or so, I believed I alone held the secret of the ashy moon until I met Bill. He not only knew about it but found it as mysterious and romantic as I did. Later, when we were married, we were flying in our plane from East Hampton to New York when Bill pointed out the cockpit window. There, a bit closer, was the ashy moon.

On this night, decades later, the ashy moon does not feel romantic; rather, it feels strangely disquieting. I close the shutters and go to bed.

In the middle of the night, I wake with a raging fever, shivering, teeth chattering, skin burning like dry ice. I fumble for the thermometer: 103°. I'm supposed to call the doctor's night number if I run a fever over 101°. I reach for the phone, but then I stop. He'll tell me to go to the ER, won't he?

I'm alone in the apartment. My last visitor, Sally, had left the Thursday before to spend Easter with her husband, Dick. Cedars is a good half-hour away. I try to force my fevered brain to think. Billy lives 20 minutes away. Do I really want to wake him? With two toddlers in the house, a night's sleep is hard to come by. The truth is the ER waiting room is the last place you want to be with or without a raging fever.

Instead, I manage to swallow two aspirins, hoping they'll stay down, and let my head fall back onto the pillow. I'd rather stay right here in my own bed and take my chances, although in my semi-delirium I am in no condition to examine what those chances might be. Then in a sudden flash of clarity I think, No, wait! I do not want to die. Not yet. Not alone in the dark. By that point I cannot even pick up the phone.

I have not been on terribly good speaking terms with God, especially since I began to see the consequences of all the free will that as far as I'm concerned he dispenses much too liberally.

The God of my childhood was different. He was the kind old

geezer sitting up on a cloudbank who used to stop the rain for me so that I could go riding. He was fair and just and always took time to listen. He could help me find things, like the time I lost the charm bracelet my father gave me for my birthday, when I turned 7, I think. Each charm represented a thing I loved: a horse, a book, an angel in ballet shoes, a tiny Aladdin's lamp.

I prayed with all my might to find it. I remember lying on my back on the floor of my bedroom, hands clasped, tears streaming into my ears, when something made me turn my head to the right. There beneath the chest of drawers, back in the dark corner next to a leg, my bracelet glittered.

My nice Geezer who took such very good care of me and of whom I was extremely fond had long gone the way of Santa Claus and the Easter Bunny. It has been hard for me to find my way to God in a world gone mad with vicious faith. One half the world intent on murdering the other half; and half of our own country hating the other half, all in the name of some version of God that I did not know and wanted nothing to do with.

I think a large part of my travels to other, older cultures was a search to reunite with the Geezer of my childhood and find a place for him in ancient teachings. Buddhists do not worship one single God. The Buddha's world, 500 years before Christ, was filled with many gods. Native Americans are both mono-theistic and pantheistic. They see the Creator in all of nature. A large rock is a grandfather, a large tree is a grandmother. The Sioux call God Wakantanka: Wakan meaning mystery, Tanka meaning great. The New-Agers, who came into being one-thou-sand, nine-hundred and sixty-eight years after Christ, pray and petition the Universe—the planets, the sun and all one sextillion stars—badgering them to grant health, love and abundance (a new car, a partner, a winning lottery ticket). I don't know, somehow I have trouble with empowering Jupiter or Saturn to save me. Since I could not find a grown-up version of my Geezer anywhere, I stopped looking.

And yet. And yet I have seen things—in Brazil and India and on the Pine Ridge Indian Reservation in South Dakota. I have glimpsed the landscape of the unseen world, which lets me know that there is something, some power far greater than the mere human mind can put a name to. The elders of the Ojibwa tribe, who named this month The Moon of the Awakening, taught: *The Great Spirit who sent sickness and death also blessed the people with the gift of healing.*

I try very hard to concentrate on this, but my body is now a block of ice. My skin burns cold. Finally, I close my eyes and try to conjure the image of my Geezer sitting up there on his cloudbank. "You probably don't remember me, God…"

Colors appear behind my eyelids and spin.

Then all goes black.

I feel nothing.

After a time, I don't know how long, whether hours or minutes, I begin to feel some sort of presence. They're here. The tree monsters —they have come for me.

Terrified, I peer into the darkness. Standing over me, big as life and plain as day, is not one of the gnarled and dwarfed creatures but a man. His eyes are kind. Somehow even in the dark I can see they are bright nut-brown. His grayish-brown hair is pulled back into a long pony tail. He is wearing a striped shirt, a soccer jerscy. His face looks Native American with high cheekbones, wide brow, arched nose, a full generous mouth. He holds both his hands above me in a gesture of healing. I keep very still. Warmth, like the radiance from one of the umbrella-like heaters used during cooler months on the patios of California restaurants, spreads over me. Not the icy burning hot of the fever but a soft, pleasant warmth that starts at my feet and flows up my legs to my abdomen, where it lingers and goes even deeper. Then, the warmth moves up into my chest and into the upper part of my body. My face is bathed in it.

Next, it is morning. White sunlight blazes at the window and floods my room. The fever's gone. The sheets are soaked. I get up and shower and dress and go for a walk. Halfway up the hill I spot a hawk circling overhead. As he veers, sunlight catches his topside and I see it is a red-tail. It is joined by another and they soar upward together, higher and higher until they are two specks in a cloudless sky. Soon, they disappear.

It is only then that I remember the shaman. There is a perfectly good explanation: fever dreams can produce images so vivid, so three dimensional that you would swear they were real. I have had fever dreams; this was not one of them. I don't know how I know this, I just know. I also know something more, something about healing I'd almost forgotten, something about my Geezer and finding the charm bracelet in the dark. I understand then in that moment what it was the dream was showing me, that I am getting help from the world way beyond the White Coats.

I walk on past the large rocks and great trees and feel the spirits alive in them and know those same spirits are alive in me, too.

The growing and dying of

the moon reminds us of our

ignorance which comes and goes

but when the moon is full it is as if

the Great Spirit was upon

the whole world.

Oglala Sioux

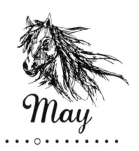

May

· · · · · o · · · · · · · ·

THE MOON WHEN THE PONIES
SHED THEIR SHAGGY HAIR

This is the part every woman dreads: the eyebrows and eyelashes go too. It is hard to be brave without eyebrows and eyelashes. The "sibs" (as Bill and I used to refer the six siblings) want to give me an expensive movie-star wig. I'm touched, but that's not what I want. An inexpensive dynel will do just fine. I find a huge wig store in the Valley, miles of wigs of every color and style for men and women. Are they all for chemo patients, I wonder? I spot a familiar face, an actress hiding behind dark glasses, trying on wigs to add to her already large hair, and a fortyish man with a thinning pate buying a curly rock-star type mop; and I feel better. Ten minutes later I walk out with a fashionably highlighted bob that at a distance in a semi-darkened room might pass for my own.

Dear Ones,

My wig is divided into six:
The perky bangs are Debbie the Dress-Up-Princess.
The glamorous wave on one side is pure Sally.

While on the other side, the wave that winds behind my ear
belongs to my spiritual (and alliterative) Wendy.
The crown belongs to Billy who ran the whole Wig Show.
The locks that hug my neck are Anthony and Mark.
Since we are such an unruly family I will take the Dress-up-
Princess' advice and head straight to a hair stylist to arrange all
these disparate locks, each of which remind me that I am loved.

Thank you, dear six,
Yr loving Mom/Sandy/Wick [short for "Wicked Stepmother"]

Another holiday. Mother's Day. (Time, slow down a bit, won't you?) Another family brunch at Billy's and HJ's. I have eliminated at least half the drugs from my routine, replacing them with vitamins, the very ones I was told not to take because it might interfere with the action of the chemo. Natural-born contrarian that I am, I have decided that they—*They*—are wrong. I need the vitamins to help rebuild my shattered, war-torn immune system. I need acidolphilus and biffidus to replace the good bacteria destroyed by the antibiotics, collateral damage. Besides, I have this new-found sense that I am protected by something I have yet to put a name to, have no need to put a name to. I am filled with a secret kind of joy that I dare not express in words for fear the spoken words might chase away this precious feeling. I smile thinking: here I sit bald as Humpty Dumpty and sitting just as precariously upon the wall, a time bomb ticking away inside me, and I've never been happier. The White-Coats would put me on one of their psycho drugs if they knew.

Everyone remarks on how well I look. I probably do look well after painstakingly applying make-up to cover the cancer pallor. It's a hue particular to cancer, I've noticed: a yellowish gray with a parchment-dry texture that I see in the faces in the waiting room of the cancer center. I've discovered that a light self-tanner works wonders and tons of moisturizer, a creamy blush, eyeliner to disguise the bald eyelids, eyebrow pencil (brushed on, for god's sake, not drawn), easy on the lipstick, then the wig, and most important, concealer for the dark circles under the eyes.

Concealing is imperative. Cancer pallor is very like a wheelchair or prosthesis: it sets you apart from everyone else. You look different; you are no longer part of the general population. You are someone who's marked for a destiny too dark to contemplate.

I try to observe people's reactions from an interested journalist's point of view: pity, which they try hard to hide; personal fear, which they really hide; and then there's the occasional genuine caring. I look around the brunch table this Mother's Day and wonder whether the love I see in my family's eyes is a bit more urgent. No need for the urgency, I want to say. I'm here right now, I'm well right now. And so very blessed.

There were other Mother's Days when I didn't feel so blessed. The years at my own mother's table when no matter how hard we tried, she and I could not reach each other. I see us straining, our fingertips slipping further and further apart. No matter how desperately we wished things were otherwise, there were always the casual words that stung, the innocent questions that rankled. Somehow long ago, at a very young age when little girls are supposed to adore their mothers, I became lost to her and she to me.

I once asked her, "When do you think we stopped understanding each other?"

"When you started having a mind of your own," was her incredible answer.

Thinking back on those days, I realize I was reaching out to her with one hand, while I was trying to hang onto my soul with the other. Years on the shrink's couch have never resolved this for me. It still makes me sad.

In 1995 when my mother turned 90, she bought me an apartment in Palm Beach, so I could be near her during her last years. What an opportunity, I thought so naively it makes me blush now to write it—to heal our wounds before it's too late. The lovely waterfront apartment she bought me was a half-hour drive away. I drove to see her twice a day, taking her shopping or to doctor's appointments or to just spend time getting to know each other in a new way.

"Where were you?"

"When?"

"You were supposed to be here an hour ago."

"No I wasn't. We said around eleven. It's eleven-fifteen."

"I wanted to go over some papers with you, now there isn't time."

"Why not? There's plenty of time. We don't have a doctor's appointment."

"That's not the point. What were you doing all morning?" Her cold eyes bore into me, and in the ninety-degree heat, I shivered.

In my early years I used to think my mother didn't love me;

and in the deepest part of me I grew up believing that somehow I must not have deserved her love, that I lacked whatever it was that make children irresistibly lovable to their mothers. I was sure it was biologically impossible for a mother not to love her child; therefore there had to be something wrong with me. She was quick to point out little things to me at various times, things I couldn't make sense of. Still, they all added up to an inchoate feeling of guilt and anxiety that in some way I was not *something* enough to deserve her love. It became clear to me finally that year in Palm Beach that it didn't matter what I did. Nothing I could do or say or be would gain me her approval. Or her love. Our hearts had already hardened against each other.

Bill came down to Florida to see me, and we talked about it. "Hey, she bought you an apartment," my psychotherapist former husband said, "She didn't buy *you*." He made frequent visits that year, so did my sons and step-daughters.

That year taught me something. It didn't remove the pain, but it did show me any rapprochement between the two of us was doomed to fail from the beginning: my mother's lack of love had nothing to do with me; it had to do with her mother's inability to love her, which had to do with her mother before that. Mother after mother, right down through the generations, all lacking the same nurturing gene and passing it on like straight hair and good skin to their daughters. I like to think that by having three sons I broke the curse. Stepdaughters, thank God, do not figure in this equation.

When his divorce was finalized, Bill moved to Albuquerque. As I had lived in Santa Fe for a while and liked it, Bill asked me if I'd consider moving back to New Mexico. I packed up, hugged my mother goodbye and wished her well.

My mother lived another five years. She died alone, except for her nurse asleep in another room, in the middle of the night the day after my last visit. Our hands and hearts never did find a way to meet.

· · · · · · · · · · · · ·

I am here now at my son's table on Mother's Day surrounded by love deeply shared, having a family favorite: shad roe sautéed in butter and served with lemon and capers and bacon (yes, bacon, dammit!) and champagne. We raise our glasses and make toasts, careful to avoid any hint of poignancy. With cancer, poignancy is not your friend.

Something in me has shifted. Whatever the spirit-shaman brought to me weeks before is still with me. The vitamins that doctors and nurses told me not to take have helped with my energy and my mood, too. When I look up at the chemo drip, I close my eyes and let myself feel the warmth from the shaman's hands spread over me. In my mind's eye I watch as he places his large hands over and around the drip, transmuting it with his alchemical powers into a precious elixir. I focus on this, shutting out all other thoughts but this one and all sounds and movements. My focus is single-pointed. I breathe deeply and allow, indeed, I welcome the images, letting them flood my body, bringing light and warmth to every cell and every mitochondria, melting the cancer cells and transmuting them into healthy, friendly cells that rejoin the rest of the harmonious population.

The chemo is liquid sunlight, or the shards of crystals that fall from the stars and planets throughout the universe and shine on the Buddha's lotus. Or the fragrance from Wakantanka's pipe. I have no nausea, much less weakness, and no fever or flu-like symptoms. I am definitely on to something here. I can barely contain my excitement. I am beginning to see what the Tibetan rimpoches in Dharamsala meant when they talked about harnessing the mind. The mind, this wondrous mind (not to be confused with the gray spongy matter inside the skull called the brain) is capable of performing miracles if we can but harness its powers. The brain powers the body, but it is the mind that powers the soul. Together there is no more powerful healing force on earth.

I am using the time between treatments to study these teachings I received that summer of 1994 to strengthen my mind. I memorized this poem from Buddha's teachings:

Know all things to be like this:
A mirage, a cloud castle,
A dream, an apparition,
Without essence, but with qualities that can be seen.

Know all things to be like this:
As the moon in a bright sky
In some clear lake reflected,
Though to that lake the moon has never moved.

Know all things to be like this:
As an echo that derives

From music, sounds, and weeping,
Yet in that echo is no melody.

Know all things to be like this:
As a magician makes illusions
Of horses, oxen, carts and other things,
Nothing is as it appears.

On the third week of this moon of the bald ponies, I have the post-chemo PET/CT tests. These will determine how I am responding to the treatments, whether and how much the tumor has shrunk and whether to continue chemo or wait and give my body a chance to recover before going another round.

I am injected with radioactive fluid, then told to lie motionless on a cold metal table while it slides into a plastic chamber. I close my eyes and dream of Brazil. I dream of the tiny village of Abadiania where I had gone to research my book, *The Brazilian Healer with the Kitchen Knife.* As the table slides in and out of the tube, I imagine myself standing in front of the man called John of God or Joao de Deus. With a quick wave of his hand (or the unsterilized kitchen knife), he removes my tumor. At the same time, he dissolves any stray cancer cells that might still be hiding in one of my lymph nodes or organs, microscopic cells that the scans cannot pick up.

I had gone to Brazil to research my book on healers from around the world. I waited in line with 200 others, Brazilians mostly, to see the man, who by channeling 34 different spirit doctors, surgeons and saints, was said to perform medical miracles. The man standing in front of me in line told me that John of God had restored his sight after five years of blindness.

"How?" I asked.

"He held my eyes open with one hand and with the other he scraped the surface with an unsterilized kitchen knife," he said.

"The surface? What surface?"

"Of my eyeballs."

The thought of that almost caused me to faint.

"I was cured of a brain tumor," another man, a Brazilian, said. "I have the X-rays. I brought them to show to Joao. See that woman standing up there? She has a tumor on her breast. Joao will remove it."

At the far end of the hall up on a stage, John of God was performing "spiritual" surgery on a woman's breast using that same unsterilized kitchen knife without anesthesia. Lifting her blouse, he made a small cut and reached in with his bare hand to remove a mass of tissue. Then, he wiped away the few drops of blood with a piece of cotton. The mass was sent to a lab in Brasilia, and the next day word came back that the tumor was found to be cancerous.

At the Casa do dom Inacio (House of Saint Ignatius), where the healings took place, was a team of physicians from England who had been observing John of God for a week. I spoke to them at the *pousada* where we were all staying. Hard as they tried, they could find no trickery, even standing right next to Joao and peering over his shoulder.

"How do you explain it then?" I asked.

"We can't. We don't even believe it. We're seeing it right in front of our eyes and we still don't believe it."

"So if it isn't trickery…" I looked from one to the other. I was writing about this; I was hoping they could offer another explanation.

"If it isn't trickery, then we're in the realm of magic and voodoo, the sort of thing that makes us extremely uncomfortable. Especially when it works."

Here I am a world away in the middle of Los Angeles, encapsulated in a 21st century positron-sensing chamber that takes pictures of the tumor that any shaman worth his salt would be able to see with the naked eye. I am on this side of the rainbow now where troubles do not melt like lemon drops, they have to be blasted to kingdom come with liquefied mustard gas.

A few days later the PET/CT report comes back: "No evidence of active disease." Doctor Quinn is amazed. And after only seven treatments! I'm thrilled too, but I'm not amazed.

I email the six siblings. "The word of the day, guys: No evidence of active disease!" I want to set that phrase to music. I also want to share what I know with my Western doctors, tell them what I have experienced firsthand—the true nature of healing. I've tried. I've given them each my book on healers, but their eyes glazed over. Unlike the British doctors who at least feel 'uncomfortable' with the mystery, my doctors' smiles are not only condescending but dismissive. I am left feeling like the eager five-year-old trying to explain to a parent the existence of fairies.

There has to be a place right here on this side of the rainbow where one day perhaps, ancient and modern, spiritual and chemical can meet and learn from each other. In the meantime it saddens me to think how many people might benefit by such a meeting.

Moon was sad. She had spent many years

looking at the people on Earth and

saw that they were afraid. They were

afraid of dying. To make them feel better she

decided to call on her friend Spider to take

a message to them. "Spider", she said, "The

people of Earth are afraid of dying and that

makes me very sad. Please tell them that they

will all die sooner or later but it is nothing

to be scared of." To this day, Spider is still

carefully carrying Moon's message and

spinning the web in the corner of our rooms —

but how many of us listen?

Cherokee Moon Legend

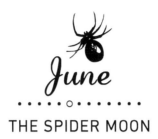

June

THE SPIDER MOON

Not so fast. Quinn wants to start me on another drug—Zometa, a bisphosphonate that in certain studies has been known to be effective in preventing bone metastasis. If there is no evidence of active disease, I ask, why worry about metastasis?

He explains that certain cancers do show up down the road in the bone, and mine is one of them. There are some side effects, he says, rare cases of necrosis (death or destruction of bone tissue) of the jaw have been reported. I nod. It's as if I've been through a reeducation program: chemo is good, chemo has saved me. Yes, of course, I want more. I know now how to control the side effects.

As I watch the nurse hook me up and I see the bag bulging with the stuff, my mind rears up like a wild horse, whinnying and pawing the air. I can't get it to stop, no matter how hard I try. My mind's gone out of control. Try as I might, I cannot capture the images I used before to create the alchemy that turned the dross dripping into my arm into liquid gold.

After the infusion I experience terrible bone and joint pain and fever. I call the office. Quinn calls back and tells me that after a few more treatments my body will adjust to the new tonic-toxin.

I have to stop my early morning walks. I can barely make it to the car to do grocery shopping, let alone cook and do my usual errands. There are no more dinners out with friends, and my visits to the boys are curtailed. My back hurts too much to lift them. My knees are too sore to even stoop to play with them. And, I can't write; my brain fog's too bad.

Four weeks later I go in for my second Zometa treatment. I am determined this time to tame the wild horse and focus on the shaman and his hands. I can do it, I tell myself. I've done it before. I know how.

The waiting room is full, standing-room only today. A nurse brings out some folding chairs, and I take the one she offers me. I have come to recognize many of the faces in the waiting room. Arranged like a large living room with couches and upholstered chairs, there's even a white upright piano with a pink breast cancer ribbon painted on it that was donated by the family of a former patient. "Former" because she was cured or "former" because she is no more, I wonder?

The space is very unlike the waiting room at Cedars, where straight-backed chairs are lined up along the walls like seats in a police station. Here at Norris, the waiting room is more conducive to conversation.

It's a strange sort of people-watching I engage in. Each of us is a citizen of the same dangerous Land of Cancer—some living perilously, some bravely, some in fear. Some will survive and get to return home to the Land of the Well; others will not. One thing is certain: none of us will ever be the same.

A man in a New York Mets cap sitting across from me looks up from his laptop, which he has duct-taped to a board. I almost don't recognize him. When I first saw him, he looked like a lumberjack, tall, ruddy, with a great bushy beard and a reddish mustache. It was only the laptop and the stack of blue-lined pages that gave him away.

Over the past few months, I have watched him shrink, lose his beard and mustache, and his complexion fade to that gray-green color of cancer.

"I've written almost a whole screenplay during these four months of chemo," he says. He grins a wry sort of grin. "Wonder if I'll ever get to find out the ending."

Another woman, hooked up to an oxygen tank, sits doing needlepoint as she talks to a little girl of about ten who is doing her homework while her mother reads a newspaper. Both the woman and the little girl are wearing yellow Live Strong bracelets. The girl's bald head is uncovered, smooth and shiny and proud in its nakedness. Her large eyes are lashless and browless, and her huge smile with a small gap between the front teeth makes me want to cry. I wonder how she'll look in the next few months. No, I don't wonder; I know.

I look at the old people with their crutches and oxygen tanks and wonder if they were that old six months ago? I want to pile them all in my car and take them to Philippe's French Dip and buy them all a triple-dip and beer and a bag of potato chips.

I recognize one woman immediately. We had both lost our hair at about the same time and showed up one day in our identical, brand new wigs, standard issue for members of the C club.

We laughed. When she saw me tugging at mine to keep it in place, she showed me something she had found at a notions store, a sticky headband to wear under the wig that serves as an anchor to keep the wig in place. When I asked, she jotted down the name of the store for me. I showed her a make-up I discovered that seemed to give a healthy glow and invited her to try some. As she brushed it on her cheeks, her cellphone rang. I remarked on the unusual ring tone.

· · · · · · · · · · · · ·

"It's a song," she said, "by Don Henley." To my blank expression, she explained, "A former Eagle."

More bewildered, I asked, "A football player?"

At that she burst into gales of laughter that set off giggles in everyone within earshot. Laughing so hard she could hardly get the words out. "No! Eagles the rock band!" Then dabbing at her eyes, she said, "It's The Heart of the Matter."

I frowned. "It is?"

That brought fresh giggles. "The title of the song. The Heart of the Matter. Listen." And she replayed the melody.

Today she looks ashen. She sits, head buried in her hands. When she looks up, her eyes are teary and swollen. I ask whether she'd like some water. She shakes her head.

"I wouldn't be able to hold it down," she says and explains that she is starting her 12th round of chemo today.

"I feel like I've been throwing up for six months straight," she says. "I'm never out of bed for more than a few hours at a time." She pauses, dabs at her eyes. "My doctor believes in going after the cancer very aggressively," she explains. "Even after the tumors have gone."

I frown, puzzled.

"Just in case."

"Just in case?" I am dumfounded. My first thought, my absolutely certain thought is that I would not be willing to do that. I don't know what I would do, only that I could not, would not go 12 rounds.

As if reading my mind, she explains that the aggressive approach is justified because hers is the kind of cancer that's almost impossible to slow down: Transitional Cell Carcinoma. Stage III.

My heart skids to a stop. It's the same diagnosis as mine. Only mine, because it had already metastasized at the time of diagnosis, is stage IV.

"It always comes back," she says. "Always."

Nervously, I look away. I am seized with an impulse to get up and leave, to flee this place that does not feel even remotely like a place of healing. I see myself stand, gather up my purse and my notebook, put on my jacket, and walk out down the hall to the double doors that lead to freedom. I see the valet take my ticket, locate my keys on his board, and trot off to get my car. But here I am, still sitting here glued to my seat. The nurse comes out, clipboard in hand, and calls out my name. I don't answer. She calls out again, louder.

"Isn't that you?" the woman next to me says.

I nod. "I suppose that is," I say and get up.

I follow her slowly, haltingly, into the treatment room. She takes my jacket and puts my purse and my notebook on the table next to the recliner, chatting on about her upcoming vacation.

"Look," I say, "I don't think I want to do this today."

"Sandra," she sings out, "You're here! Don't be silly. Do you know how lucky you are?" She hangs the IV bag and unfolds the tubing. "I have to take this drug by mouth once a month because I couldn't possibly afford the IV. In four treatments you get all the dosage you need for a year. I take it as a preventive against bone loss and I've never had cancer. Believe me, this is a miracle drug. You're lucky to have insurance. Do you know what each treatment costs? Close to a thousand dollars!"

Dr. Quinn walks by. "Hi! How's the writing going?" he asks cheerily. "When you gonna finish that book?"

I am a coward. I settle into the recliner and open the top two buttons of my shirt to allow access to the shunt.

"Labs looking good," Quinn says as he walks on.

I lack the courage to stand up for what I know to be true. By the way, the name is Sandy, not Sandra. Big deal. I'm a fraud.

· · · · · · · · · · · · ·

The second Zometa treatment is worse than the first. The reaction lasts longer: flu symptoms, joint and back pain. My white blood cell counts have fallen so low that I can't be around Billy and Danny if they have even a sniffle; and, toddlers, notorious germ machines that they are, always have a sniffle. I'm warned that a simple cold virus could eventually land me in the hospital with pneumonia.

When I look up the drug Zometa on the Internet, I notice along the right hand side of the screen a list of law firms offering to represent patients suffering from jaw osteonecrosis (also known as dead jaw) linked to Zometa. Big law firms suing big pharmaceutical companies. New Mercedes Benzes for all. The chemo nurse was right: a thousand bucks a pop. That's on top of the cost of chemo, which can run over a hundred thousand dollars, up 15 percent from the year before. I read on. There's a warning: *Patients with kidney disease may not be candidates for bisphosphonate therapy and should discuss their condition with their physician.*

Hold on. Wait a minute. Isn't the tumor we're trying to shrink *inside* the kidney?

The question rages on inside my head. What *if?* What if, as the woman in the waiting room said, it always does, it comes back? I had thought before this diagnosis and after my bout with breast cancer 15 years before that if I ever had a recurrence, my self-treatment would be carrots, broccoli, asparagus and juices, herbs and vitamins; and I would seek out the best healers on the planet. I said that, I believed that with all my heart. Then the worst happened, and the mind stopped, frozen.

It's like coming up against a mugger on a dark street holding a gun. You don't stop to ponder the alternatives. You give him your wallet and ask whether he wants your watch and your ring, too. You just want to live. Your family wants you to live. The consensus is that if you want to live, you take your medicine and don't ask questions. The consensus is never wrong, is it?

The eternal/internal debate continues: at night when I'm trying to settle in with a good book, afternoons when I'm with the little boys, mornings when I am able to take my walks again. The pharmaceutical companies will always come out with new drugs with new side effects. Why call them *side* effects? They're not side effects at all; they are the drug's *effects*.

Look, I argue, I beat cancer before with chemo, and I'm beating it again now. What is my problem? My problem is, I argue back, that I never really did beat it the first time. If I had, it wouldn't have come back 15 years later. And what about my annual Christmas cold, my springtime flu and the summer bronchitis that lasts into fall? Are these not the results of a compromised immune system? This is the underlying problem, I conclude. The civil war inside my head rages on.

I make an appointment to see Dr. Agre and ask him about the Zometa. To my surprise, he agrees. He is aware of the statistics on kidney problems resulting from the drug and doesn't like it. "Don't take it," he advises.

At my next scheduled appointment for lab tests and a brief consult with Quinn, I tell him of my decision and that Keith Agre backs me up.

"Those numbers are rare," he says, but based on the reaction I'm having, he agrees I might be one of the few people who do not tolerate bisphosphonates well.

It has taken me the rest of this Spider Moon, but I have finally snapped myself out it. There was a very good reason I couldn't turn that particular dross to gold: for my body it was dross. My mind, my wondrous mind, knew it.

When the buffalo are fat,

When new sprouts of sage are a span long,

When chokecherries are ripening,

When the Moon is rising

as the Sun is going down,

That is the time for the Sacred Sun Dance.

Lakota Sioux

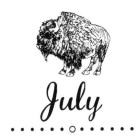

July
· · · · · · ○ · · · · · ·

THE MOON OF THE SACRED SUNDANCE

In this hot summer month, everyone seems to be away. Billy and HJ have taken the children back east to the beach. Friends all seem to be off somewhere. Even my doctors are away. A temporary cease fire is in effect—I have stopped thinking about tests and treatments. Without the Zometa, my joint pains are gone and the brain fog's cleared. I can concentrate now on the reconstruction of my immune system. First, clear out the toxins. I go to the farmer's market and stock up on fresh vegetables and fruits. Just down the street is a health food store that makes fresh juices. Each day I try a new combination: apple, celery, beet and carrot one day; a green juice another. I switch from coffee to tea, from sugar to honey, eat less meat, more fish, and drink lots and lots of water.

Detoxing my mind comes next. Afternoons when the shadows are long and the air is cool, I walk a bit farther up the hill behind my house, a spiral notebook tucked under my arm. There's a bench near the top of the hill where I can sit and do my scribbling. I've started keeping a journal to track this strange journey

I've found myself on. I can count 22 countries I've traveled to in as many years. Now I can add another: the Land of Cancer, which is cold and barren and war-torn, like Iraq in winter. I'm getting up at dawn and writing five pages a day. I must write myself well. Writing's my medicine, the real alchemy that stabilizes all the unstable elements and heals the soul. It is the best way I know to find my way home.

A hummingbird hovers near me at eye level for a moment then heads for a small sapling that I had not noticed before and perches on a tiny, fragile branch. On the branch below hangs a small scrap of red cloth that had probably gotten caught on it. I let my gaze rest on it as it flutters in the breeze. It reminds me of the prayer flags of both the Tibetan and the Native American rituals so much a part of their daily lives. I remembered Hopi spiritual leader, Martin Gashweseoma, explaining to me that if you dropped a plumb line from Hopi in Arizona through the center of the earth, it would come out at the holy city of Lhasa in Tibet. The similarities do not end there. The words for sun and moon in Tibetan and Hopi are the same but reversed. Many of both peoples' chants and symbols are similar, including the use of prayer flags to carry blessings on the wind.

I'm thinking of another July in 1992, just months after I finished treatments for breast cancer. I remember a tall cotton-wood in the center of the Sun Dance grounds on the Pine Ridge Indian Reservation in South Dakota with red, blue, green and white pieces of cloth fluttering from its bare branches. The Lakota Sioux called them offering flags.

I had driven to Pine Ridge from Santa Fe that morning as

part of my research for *The Book of Elders: Stories & Wisdom of Great American Indians*. Pete Catches, holy man of the Lakota Sioux and a man I had come to call "Grandfather", had invited me to witness the most sacred of all Lakota rituals, the Sun Dance.

The dancers, pledgers they were called, had each been pierced with small eagle bones on each side of their chests by the medicine man. The eagle bone skewers were then fastened to the top of the tree by a long rope.

"This sacred cottonwood tree represents the center of the world," Catches explained. "It connects the heavens to the earth. The dancers must show bravery, endurance, and integrity to be granted their sacred dream, their vision."

At a signal from the medicine man, the pledgers began to circle the tree to the sound of beating drums. I can still hear the sounds of those whistles and rattles, and the dancers feet pounding the bare ground. Then, one by one, the dancers began to yank backward, four times, with all their strength, until the skewers were torn loose and with them a piece of their flesh. These pieces of flesh were placed at the foot of the tree as offerings. Members of the tribe were deep in prayer, their benedictions a spiritual wind that swept over the entire Sun Dance grounds. The pledgers and the tribe were then free to seek their vision.

I was so deeply engrossed that I did not notice the young man approach, not until he tapped me on the shoulder.

"Grandfather wants you to come stand in the arbor," he said in a hushed, reverential voice.

At first I did not understand.

"Come with me," the boy said.

I followed him to an opening in the circle where an arbor stood, decorated with boughs of sage and cedar and red, green, blue and white prayer flags. The boy pointed to the arbor, indicating that I was supposed to stand there. A moment later, to the sounds of rattles and song, Pete Catches came toward me, a large eagle feather in his hand. He sang out a prayer as he swept the feather over and around me. Tears spilled down my cheeks and dried on my face in the hot breeze. "Go live your dream now," he said.

That day marked an opening for me into the unseen world. I saw with striking clarity the power of spiritual forces at work. I believe that blessing kept me well for 15 years. Perhaps, in some way I have yet to understand, it still is protecting me.

On this July day a decade and a half later, I look up at the sun and try to hold its furious glare for a few seconds. So far I have charted my course by the changing face of the moon. Now, in this month of the Sun Dance when the chokecherries are ripe and the moon rises while the sun is still in the sky, it is the sun that speaks to me. It asks if this is not the time to reassess the power of the spiritual forces I once saw with such clarity that day on the Sun Dance grounds. To see again how I have been guided and protected, even through my recent brush with mortality. Most of all, it asks me, "Are you living your dream?"

I think about the stone carver sitting by the side of the road under a makeshift tent in Dharamsala. His few belongings—a cup, a bowl, some candles, sticks of incense, bottles of water—were neatly arranged to one side. On the other, stacks of

99

scriptures lovingly wrapped in cloth sat next to piles of smooth stones. I stopped to watch as he carved a mantra onto a stone, so deep in concentration he did not notice me. Through a translator I asked him what he was going to do with the stones. He explained that he puts them on the top of a hill near the river. The water that touches the stones spreads the blessings carved on them. The wind that blows across the stones saves insects and all living things from a bad rebirth. "In the morning I burn three incense sticks and pray that whatever merit I accumulate carving these stones may be for the benefit of all sentient beings."

My gaze falls on the little sapling with the scrap of red cloth hanging from it. Like the stone-carver, I carve my dreams upon the page and let the wind do the rest. This is my pledge.

The Kachina (spirit beings) came to the Hopi people long ago in an ancient village in a time of drought and starvation. The people began to die. When all hope was lost, the Kachina saw the people's suffering and took pity on them. They materialized in human-like form to help them with their power to grow food, bring rain and heal the sick through prayers of song and dance. The word Kachina means "life bringer." Twice a year, in August, and again in February for the winter solstice, the Kachina appear to the Hopi to bless the people, to bring rain and bountiful harvest, and to heal the sick. On the full moon, the Flute Clan conducts its dances. The people are joyful.

Hopi

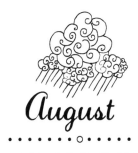

August

. . . . o . . . . .

THE MOON OF THE JOYFUL

During the first week of this Moon of the Joyful, I come through another PET/CT scan with flying colors. Both my red and white blood cell counts are normal for the first time since I began chemo. The alert level has been lowered to green; I can stop worrying about germs. I spend more time with the little ones, go out to restaurants, and to a crowded movie theatre where people actually cough and sneeze and I do not get pneumonia. I can even get on an airplane. Funny how I don't seem to mind the long lines, or the scowling security lady who barks at me to throw away my water bottle. I don't even mind the kid who's seated behind me and keeps kicking the back of my seat. I'm flying to Albuquerque to see my youngest son, Anthony (whose birthday is on the 13th) and his two boys, five-year-old AJ and three-year-old Alec.

I am back in the Land of the Well, where people grumble about flight delays and shout into their cell phones and eat junk food from airport kiosks. They stare with blank expressions at the TV screen above their heads or read newspapers or thumb their Blackberries. A few read books; I strain to see the titles. I want to know who these people are, living here in the Land of the Well. Do they know how lucky they are? I scan the faces, trying to pick out any who are awake to the preciousness of life. When I spot one, I smile, and they smile back.

We are flying over Arizona. I look out the window and try to pick out the pink-gray sandstone mesas of the Hopi Reservation as we near the Four Corners. I remember that trip. Barely a month after Sun Dance, I headed for Hopi territory to observe the summer Kachina ceremonies for a chapter in *The Book of Elders*. I invited a friend and student of Hopi culture, Ingrid Nelson, to make the trip with me.

We arrived at the Hopi reservation at sunset. In the shifting light and deepening shadows, the carvings on the canyon walls sprang to life; and I could feel the presence of the wind spirits. Was I sufficiently aware then of how privileged I was to be writing a book that would bring me into these worlds, and to be invited into the home of Martin Gashweseoma, keeper of the sacred stone tablets that contain the Hopi prophecy? It was as if I had traveled back in time. I marvel at how fortunate, how very blessed I was to walk with these timeless and magical beings.

I can still see Martin's white hair pulled back in a long pony tail, his face etched deep by time and wisdom. I can still taste the strong Indian coffee we drank in his kitchen, and the *piki*, a crisp and flaky corn bread baked on a stone in the traditional way. I remember hastily scribbling his words (he would not permit my tape recorder) as he spoke of the dire warnings of the prophecy. "The time of purification would come when the people would become lazy and stop walking. People would float around without their feet ever touching the ground (cars). There would be a highway in the sky (airplanes). People would look into a window to find out what was going on in the world (television). That time has come now," he said.

"Sickness, starvation, homelessness, disease and destruction of the planet are all part of the prophecy. We have to wake up right now. Stop all the wrongdoing and get balanced. If we don't stop and look at what we are doing to the planet and to the rest of the world's peoples," he warned, "there will be terrible disasters. We have no business destroying any other life."

I am reminded of these dire warnings now and how each of these prophecies has come to pass: 9/11, wars, student massacres, systematic despoiling of our environment, abandoned children, rising cancer epidemic. When I asked Martin if the time of Purification was near, he answered that we've already gone over the time limit that was given to us in the Prophecies. Those who are ready and who have a big heart will survive, but they will be tested. "Wake up right now!" he said, looking straight at me.

I listened. I wrote it all down and included his warnings in the book, but I now realize I hadn't woken up. I was there as an interested journalist. When I was tested, I failed. I watched stunned and enraged as my world began to collapse. In 1998 on Pearl Harbor Day, Bill took his own life and the moon went dark. Forever, I feared.

Three years later on September 10, 2001 friends and I gathered at a restaurant in Venice, California, to celebrate my birthday. The next day the world went crazy. Innocence, and for many, faith in the inherent goodness of man was hijacked.

A year later, one day before my mother died, people around her got her to change her will, hijacking it when she was barely coherent and had to scrawl an X for her signature, and the structure my future was built on came tumbling down.

Soon after that, our Constitution was hijacked by our own home-grown forces of darkness, and it seemed our whole democracy had been deconstructed. I worry for my children and grandchildren; I worry that as a people we still cannot, will not heed the Hopi Prophecies.

Fear and rage consumed me during those years, flowed through me just like the poison the Tibetan astrologer saw written in my stars. I wonder: was this the bitter poison that would eventually manifest itself as cancer?

· · · · · · · · · · · ·

Anthony meets me at the airport. He's handsome, smiling, and he hugs me tightly.

The New Mexico sky is crystalline, the Sangre de Christos rise emphatically to the west; at sunset, as their name promises, they will turn blood red. In the car I study my son's fine profile outlined against the New Mexico sky and feel a fresh twinge of pain when I notice its similarity to his father's.

Albuquerque is at 6,000 feet. I'd forgotten that it takes a bit of acclimatizing for someone coming from sea level. I feel the elevation as we climb the two flights of stairs to his new bachelor digs (Anthony's recently separated. God, don't let him follow in my footsteps). Later, when we pick up the children and take them to a playground and I push them on the swings and catch them on the slides, I feel the lack of oxygen even more.

I drink more water. Santa Fe, where I had lived for nine years, is another thousand feet high in elevation; but one's body has no memory. It still takes re-acclimation. I want to see Santa Fe again, drive past my old house and have lunch at my favorite restaurant. When I start to feel dizzy and headachy, when my heart begins to pound and my mouth goes dry, I attribute my condition to the altitude and force myself to drink still more water.

By Sunday when Anthony drives me to the airport, I'm having a hard time hiding my discomfort. I don't want him to wonder if my symptoms, after three whole days, have anything to do with the altitude, and I don't want him spreading the word to the sibs I seemed unwell. There is, of course, a third reason, one I don't want to think about—that it may not be altitude sickness at all.

I drag myself onto the airplane and collapse into my aisle seat and try to shove my carry-on underneath the seat in front of me. The few things I bought in Santa Fe have caused the bag to bulge at the seams. I get up and try instead to maneuver it into the overhead. The man in the window seat next to me jumps to his feet and helps me. I laugh, embarrassed, and thank him. He smiles back. He's silver-haired, tanned, well-dressed, fit. Everything about him reminds me of every man I've ever been attracted to.

He strikes up a conversation. We fall into easy talk about the balloons in the distance, which are probably practicing for Albuquerque's annual hot-air balloon fest coming up in October. Have I ever been up in a balloon? Yes, it was pretty bumpy, windy that day. You? Yes, once in Switzerland. Over the Alps? Yes, it was spectacular.

The conversation turns to flying. He got his private license 20 years ago. I got mine about the same time. Really, where? East Hampton. You? Teterboro. In a Piper Cub. I got mine in a Cessna 150. (He's not wearing a ring, I notice.) Where do you live? I live in Los Angeles now, but I used to live in New York. (His smile is intimate.) Me too. I lived in New York for 25 years, but after my wife passed away I moved to Newport. Now I sail instead of fly. Do you still fly? No, not for years. His eyes are warm, intelligent, and frankly admiring. I wonder if we're going to exchange business cards.

After several moments in which neither of us speaks, I take out the book I'm reading, *The Biology of Belief: Unleashing the Power of Consciousness, Matter and Miracles* by Dr. Bruce Lipton, and open to a page I had marked with a highlight pen.

"Are you a teacher?" he asks.

"I have taught creative writing, but I'm researching a book I'm writing now."

"On what?"

"Healing and healers. This is by a former medical school professor and research scientist. It's fascinating." I show him the book. He takes it and reads the back cover.

"Hmm. 'Stunning new scientific discoveries about the biochemical effects of the brain's functioning show that all the cells of your body are affected by your thoughts.' What's this got to do with healing? How does a *healer* change your thoughts?"

"A healer doesn't change your thoughts," I explain. "What the author is saying is that illness results from disturbances in one's energy fields. What a healer does is remove those disturbances or energy blocks so that mind, body and emotions flow freely and bring the body back into balance."

I stop. He is watching me with an expression I know so well.

"You believe this?" he asks with an edge to his voice.

"It's all energy," I say.

His gaze is no longer warm.

"My wife died a long agonizing death of breast cancer a year ago," he says. "Our daughter talked her into going to see an alternative doctor in New York who wanted her take about 50 different vitamins a day and shots of God knows what. She tried it for a few weeks then gave up. Then our daughter said she knew of an incredible healer who has cured cancer. My wife gave in, and we drove up to Taos to see him. The guy charged a thousand dollars a session and said that my wife would need at least six sessions, maybe more. When I questioned the fee, the bastard asked me what I thought my wife's life was worth."

He stops a moment to get his anger under control. "Are these the 'healers' you write about?"

"I make it a point never to write about healers who charge exorbitant fees," I answer.

I know this person; I have met him many times. I've even fallen in love with this person only to discover we disagree on everything from politics to art to books, and finally on the way we see each other. I also realize that his attitude on health and healing typifies that of many who feel safer in the hands of conventional modern medicine and who will defend it even if it kills them.

He reaches down and takes *The Wall Street Journal* out of his briefcase. My headache, which had mysteriously vanished, comes pounding back.

· · · · · · · · · · · · ·

Back at sea level in L.A., I expect my altitude symptoms to disappear. They don't. I'm still weak and achy, and my head feels like it's packed with cotton. I try to work. I force myself to work. Keep writing, I tell myself. Write past the headache, focus on the words and the dizziness will pass. Slip back into the story and let it envelop me, take me into its world. Breathe the fragrance of Brazil, the sea air that mingles with the pungent perfume of nutmeg and cinnamon rising from the jungles and forests. Call on the spirits that ride in on the morning mist to whisper their secrets. This is where I am always safe, in this world that I and I alone am the author of.

Are the gods the authors of our fate? Or as the popular notion insists, do we ourselves choose our own fate?

Sandy Johnson

The crops are ready for gathering. Corn, pumpkins, squash, beans, wild rice, turnips and beets. The full moon rises as the sun sets and hangs low in the sky, bringing extra light to the people who work late into the night to bring in the year's harvest. For they know it is the end of the growing season.

Zuni

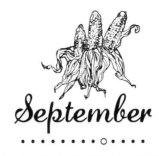

September
· · · · · · · · · ○ · · · ·
THE MOON OF CHANGE

It is a time of reflection in the dwindling summer heat, as autumn approaches. How much can I really with my mind, with meditation and a shift in my thinking affect a change in the outcome of this illness? Or is my destiny entirely in the hands of the White Coats? Doubts begin to nudge out the beliefs I cling to for dear life as I notice that three days later I'm still achy and weak, my head's still throbbing.

I have no appetite, and I'm running a slight fever. My muscles are terribly sore. I want to think it's a delayed reaction to chemo or maybe the Zometa, exacerbated by the sudden change of altitude or that maybe I'm coming down with something I picked up on the flight to New Mexico that my body is trying to fight off. I'm sleeping ten hours a night and waking up exhausted from vivid dreams that speak of danger.

I have an appointment at Norris for routine lab tests that are done every four weeks. I could ask to see Dr. Quinn, but I don't. I don't call Agre either. I have to hang onto those other possibilities. I have to, because with every fiber of my being, every shred of my will, I do not want to go back to that place, I do not want to walk again those cold and lonely halls of the Land of the Ill.

. . . .

This Moon of Change is also the month of my birth. According to the *Farmer's Almanac*, the full moon, which happens to fall exactly on my birthday, will be the brightest full moon of the whole year. I take this as a good omen.

Billy and HJ have planned another birthday dinner. Even though it's not one that's a multiple of five or ten, it's another kind of milestone: I'll be there to celebrate it. The party turns out to be one of their extravagances: 20 of us at a long candlelit table, beautifully laid, and set up on the patio beneath that startlingly bright moon. Tiny white lights are strung from the trees overhead. The perfect setting for the award-winning performance I'm going to have to give after the news I received the morning before.

I was on my way home from the dry cleaners, where I was picking up the outfit I planned to wear for my birthday dinner, when my cellphone rang. I was surprised to hear Dr. Quinn's voice. He was calling from the airport, he said in his broad Australian drawl, and about to board a flight to Shanghai to attend a conference. I propped the phone to my ear with my shoulder as I attempted a left turn at an intersection. I had to swerve suddenly to avoid a car that was coming from the opposite direction and the phone toppled to the floor. When I managed to retrieve it, he was saying something about my labs.

"Sorry?" I said.

"I had a chance to look at your labs before I left," he repeated. "Your liver enzymes are quite high. I'm not all that concerned, but

I think you should have Agre check them again."

I pulled over to the curb and came to a screeching halt. "…as soon as possible," he added. "I've faxed him the reports."

I sat there a moment, horns blasting at me.

The alert level just shot back up to orange.

It always comes back, the woman in the waiting room at Norris said.

But so soon? And in the liver?

What else did she say? There was something else she said, something I didn't want to remember. Oh yes. *And when it does, it comes back fast and hard.* I couldn't remember her name either—Felicia or Lena?

My heart pounded. Butterflies began to bang around in the pit of my stomach. A flame is what they're called. A swarm of butterflies is called a flame. The flame rose up from my stomach into my throat.

As soon as I got home, I put down my things and sat in a straight-backed chair to meditate. Follow the breath, I said, in and out, in and out. Still the mind and the body will follow. Buddhists call it the monkey mind when it won't hold still. Mine is a wild horse who rears up and paws frantically at the air. That morning the horse galloped away, leaving me to my burning butterflies.

I start over. I must gain control of my mind lest the butterflies release the fear hormones, the flight or fight hormones that alert the 50 trillion cells to impending danger. I need to convince those cells that there are no threats so that the hormones will quiet down and do their job of protecting the immune system and promoting life-sustaining growth.

A mantra, I need a mantra. I tried OHM. That helped for a few minutes but then the OHM turned into the whinnying of the wild horse. What about *Om mani padme hum*? A Tibetan rimpoche once told me that all the teachings of the Buddha are contained in this mantra, but that the meaning could be summed up as The True Sound of Truth. I always had trouble getting the exact pronunciation and stumbled over it now.

My mind jumps to the wonderful old story that same rimpoche told of the devoted meditator, who after years of concentrating on a particular mantra, had attained enough insight to begin teaching. His humility was far from perfect, though. A few years of successful teaching had left the meditator with no thoughts about ever learning anything more from anyone. Then one day he heard about a famous hermit who lived nearby all alone on an island at the middle of a lake. The meditator hired a man with a boat to row him across to the island.

As they shared some tea, the meditator asked the hermit about his spiritual practice. The old man said he had no spiritual practice, only a mantra which he kept repeating to himself. The meditator was pleased, as the mantra the hermit was using was the same mantra he himself used, except that when the hermit spoke the mantra aloud, the meditator gasped.

"What's wrong?" asked the hermit.

"I don't know what to say. I'm afraid you've wasted your whole life! You are pronouncing the mantra *incorrectly!*"

"Oh, dear! That is terrible. How should I say it?"

The meditator gave him the correct pronunciation, and the

old hermit was very grateful, asking to be left alone so he could get started right away. On the way back across the lake, the meditator, now satisfied that he was an accomplished teacher, pondered the sad fate of the hermit. "It's so fortunate that I came along. At least he will have a little time to practice correctly before he dies." Just then, the meditator noticed that the boatman was looking past him quite shocked at something he was seeing, and he turned to see what it was the boatman was staring at.

The hermit was standing respectfully *on the water*, next to the boat. "Excuse me, please," he said. "I hate to bother you, but I've forgotten the correct pronunciation again. Would you please repeat it for me?"

"I—I," stammered the meditator.

The old hermit persisted in his polite request until the meditator relented and told him again the way the mantra was supposed to be pronounced.

"Thank you," he said and turned and walked across the surface of the water back to the island repeating the mantra very carefully, slowly, over and over.

. . . .

I continued on with my meditation not worrying about the pronunciation or how many thoughts flitted through my mind. Finally, the wild horse exhausted itself and quieted down, and I could concentrate on cooling down the butterflies. After twenty or thirty minutes, they folded their wings.

My mind was calm enough now to place the call to Agre's office. I got a recording. Right, Saturday, the office is closed. It will be open again Monday, unless it's an emergency. No, no emergency. Definitely not an emergency. I left a message to call me Monday. I once tried to tell Dr. Agre how meditation helped me get through some very scary times, and he nodded and listened and changed the subject. Perhaps if I could actually show him how meditation caused my enzymes to return to normal, he'd take notice.

That same afternoon Agre's colleague, Dr. Chung, returned my call. He explained he was covering for Agre, who's away for a week. I told Dr. Chung about the liver enzymes. He had already seen the fax. "It could be nothing more than a mild virus," he said in a reassuring voice. "How have you been feeling?"

I mentioned my trip to New Mexico and my difficulty with the higher elevation. "Other than that," I said, "I'm feeling fine."

"You'd better come in," he said, and scheduled me for a lab test first thing Monday. First the birthday dinner.

· · · · · · · · · · · · ·

Billy and HJ had gone to great lengths to make one of my favorite dishes for the birthday dinner, but for the life of me I can't remember which one—osso bucco, maybe, or Billy's World's Best Chicken with a splendid wine and a great cake, probably from La Brea Bakery. The reason I can't remember is because it took all of my energy to stay focused on the conversation, to keep smiling until my cheeks began to hurt. Now and then the buzz of conversation would fade into the distance, or sound as if were coming from under water. I thought my performance was fine until I spotted Billy eyeing me from the other end of the table.

"What's up?" he asked sotto voce as he made his way to where I was sitting.

"Nothing really," I said. When he kept looking at me, I added quickly, "Something a little weird about my liver enzymes."

He frowned.

"I'm seeing about it tomorrow. Not to worry."

His eyes remained fixed on me a moment more. Then, lips pressed together, he took the drink I was holding out of my hand.

· · · · · · · · · · · ·

Monday morning I go to Agre's office to have the liver enzymes checked. Tuesday Dr. Chung calls back. They're still high, through the roof high. Hepatitis has been ruled out. Dr. Chung says it could be some other inflammation of the liver: a virus, perhaps, that will run its course and clear itself up in a day or two. He wants to wait a week, then run another test. Agre will be back by then and so will Quinn.

A week?

When Billy calls to ask for news, I repeat this information to him as casually as I can. I do not tell anyone else. First, I don't want to go sounding the alarm whenever anything goes wrong. One can safely assume that with cancer things go wrong fairly frequently. Second, saying something makes it too real (the rule of concretization). Not saying something leaves it in the realm of infinite possibilities.

This is the nuttiness of cancer.

How shall I spend the week? Go to Paris, stay at the Raphael, visit one of my favorite small museums, the Musée Guimet of Asian Art, and afterward have oysters on the half shell at Le Petit Zinc? Or stay home and eat potato chips? Read Proust (while eating potato chips)? See some movies? (There's a couple I really wanted to see.) Hike up the hill and sit on my bench and wait to be enlightened? Om mani padme hum.

I don't do any of these things. Instead, I stick to my routine. I pick Billy and Danny up at school and take them to Larchmont for Jamba Juice, and then to the bookstore where they each pick out a new book. Next, I go to the hairdresser. My hair has begun to come back, a good three inches now, but a ghastly brown mixed with (Oh no!) *gray*. I want my blond hair back, no matter how short. I do laundry, pay bills. I open the notice from *The New Yorker*, informing me that my subscription is ready to expire. Renew now, it says, or you won't receive the next issue. Renew for two years and you'll save another five dollars.

I stare at the notice for a long time, remembering Bill and the postage stamps. He was sitting at his desk paying bills. I was about to go shopping and asked him if he needed anything. "*Stamps*," he scrawled on his child's magic erasing pad.

"A roll?"

"*No. A sheet.*"

"That's silly. That's only 20. I'll get you a roll."

"*No. Just a sheet.*"

Because the next day he would be leaving. He was already planning it. He would take *The New York Times* into the garage and sit in the car and read it with the ignition on and wait for death. Why waste money on stamps he would never use?

I wrote out a check to *The New Yorker* to renew my subscription. For one year.

A week can fly by in a flash, barely noticed, not much remembered. I decided that instead of watching television or having long idle telephone conversations or reading the newspapers cover to cover, I could stretch the days and nights by filling them with meaningful moments—do only that which holds me happily captive to the world.

I call a friend and we get tickets to the Philharmonic to hear Ravel's Mother Goose Suite. I walk as much as I can, paying extra attention to the changing colors of the leaves (autumn does come to Southern California, and we even have a quaking aspen on our corner); I read. I go the library and take out the books I always meant to read but never got around to. I never read all four sections of William Faulkner's *The Sound and the Fury*. I couldn't get past the section on Benji. I read Colette's *Cheri* but never got around to *The Last of Cheri*.

I pick up the little boys at Pre-K and take them to Larchmont or to the corner Mexican restaurant for horchetta, a sweet rice drink they like. I eat my favorite foods with my favorite friends at my favorite restaurants and pay very close attention to what is going in their lives.

And I write. Or try to. I can't seem to keep focused on the parallel world of mine that is so precious to me.

I call my friend, Judith Prager, who's an author, therapist, and instructor at UCLA's writing program. She has been there for me since the day of the diagnosis, always ready to listen, always encouraging me both with my healing and my writing. She and her husband, poet Harry Youtt, have read a couple of drafts of the novel, and their feedback has been invaluable.

I start by telling her I'm having trouble concentrating on the novel, but at her probing I end up confessing my fear of possible liver cancer. I tell her that if I'm going to be terminally sick I want my last words to be the ones I put on the page.

"But I can't seem to write," I tell her. "I can't seem to keep my mind on the story. I'm not sure I know the ending anymore."

"Has it occurred to you that maybe at this particular moment it's another book you should be writing?" Judith replied. "I mean, aren't you living the most important story of your life? Harry and I have both wondered why you're not writing that." She asks whether I've been keeping a journal.

"Well, my scribblings, yes."

I finally admit that lately these scribblings had been demanding more and more of my writing time, like a bothersome child tugging at my sleeve while I'm sitting there sweating over the novel.

"Hmm," Judith mused. "Books demanding to be written. The gall."

Harry gets on the phone and chimes in. "Those voices in our heads deserve to be listened to," he says.

Judith adds, "You must tell your story; tell us how you found your courage."

"But I haven't found my courage," I answer. "I'm still looking."

"Then take us with you on your quest," Judith says. "Let us see what helps and what doesn't."

I think about that. For just one week, I decide to leave my protagonists Peter and Sara and the dark happenings in Brazil and turn to *Me*, my life inside the tangle that I'm figuring out how to unravel, day by day, moon by moon.

What helps? Knowledge helps. Meditation helps. What

doesn't? People who come at me with tragic faces don't help. Doctors who talk about percentages don't help. Most of all, my doubts about chemo do not help at all.

It's becoming clear to me that the problem with modern Western medicine is that it can only step in after it's too late, after the renegade cells have become a detectable tumor, after the damage has already been done. Then, the White Coats can go in and bomb the hell out of them. It's like having George Bush in control. The ancients, on the other hand, knew one must look for the cause of the illness and root it out, not just treat the symptoms with medicines that destroy but do not heal.

True to my decision back in March to defy the doctors' warnings about vitamins and other supplements, I continue to scour the Internet looking for information on how to build up my immune system. I spend hours making notes, fact-checking; I am a fiend for information. I hunt for statistics; I read up on signs and symptoms to watch for. Then, armed with my own research, I drive the doctors crazy with questions.

Poor Dr. Quinn. I quiz him about the statistics I've just read. "And what if I go past seven years? Ten? Fifteen?" Finally, I get the answer I'm looking for.

"After that," he says with a shrug, "if you make it past then, forever."

I am back in the saddle now, trotting at a fast clip across territory I know well.

I read books on beating cancer, living with cancer, dying with cancer. Even one that says cancer is not a disease at all, that cancer cells occur between six to more than ten times in a person's lifetime. If the immune system is strong, the cancer cells will die their own death (apoptosis); and, therefore, they will be prevented from multiplying and forming tumors. Patrick Quillin in his book, *Beating Cancer with Nutrition*, explains: "It is simple to kill all the cancer cells in your body. A thimble full of arsenic will do the job. The cancer cells have been killed—and so has the cancer patient. Not much of a victory."

Later, Quillin recasts his analogy to vivid effect: "…If you had mice in your garage and you used a hand grenade to blow up the garage," he writes, "then you no longer have a mouse problem, nor do you have a garage."

According to Quillin, a healthy adult body has about 60 trillion cells of which a third, 20 trillion, are immune factors. A million cancer cells are undetectable by even the most sensitive medical equipment; a billion cancer cells become a tiny, nearly undetectable lump. The crucial missing link in most cancer therapy is a way to stimulate the patient's own healing abilities to prevent a recurrence. "Imagine leaving behind only one million dandelion seeds on your lawn after you thought you got them all," Quillin writes.

In their book, *The China Study*, T. Colin Campbell and Thomas M. Campbell II explain the situation another way: "Cancer proceeds through three stages: initiation, promotion and progression…" The Campbells also use a landscape-related metaphor: "…The process is similar to planting a lawn. Initiation is when you put the seeds in the soil, promotion is when the grass starts to grow and progression is when the grass gets completely out of control, invading the driveway, the shrubbery and the sidewalk."

Dr. Andrew Weil, in his book, *Spontaneous Healing*, writes: "Healing is an inherent capacity of life. DNA has within it all the information needed to manufacture enzymes to repair itself. The healing system operates continuously and is always on call. Healing is spontaneous..."

I come up with my own metaphor. In the dark crevices and caves throughout my body, homegrown terrorist cells hide out, waiting to strike. I send them messages: "You bastards pulled a sneak attack on me, so I retaliated and bombed the crap out of you. Talk about shock and awe. Can we call a truce now?" Maybe this conflict can be resolved diplomatically. Or simply with the power of my mind.

Cell biologist Bruce Lipton talks about how our beliefs (perceptions) affect our cells. Our belief about our disease will determine the course of the disease. The trick is to determine how exactly do we change the perceptions drummed into our heads by doctors, newspapers, TV, indeed, the entire consciousness of our society that a diagnosis of advanced-stage cancer is a death sentence?

In the startling brightness of the September moon, I begin to dig into my remembered past, tilling that soil. Buried deep beneath what we think we know about the true meaning of healing lays the wisdom and knowledge of the ancients.

For instance, Tibetan Buddhists believe that illnesses like cancer can be a warning to remind us that we have been neglecting deep aspects of our being, our spiritual needs. If I am to get bad news next week, I'm going to have to call on that wisdom.

I make a renewed determination to meditate more. One hour at least. I sit, I try, I fail. I've mastered it before; I can master it again. Just say the mantra. Then, the phone rings, a shopping list pops into my head, the hammering and sawing in the apartment across the hall where my neighbors are renovating their kitchen infuriates me. I have to pee. I can't decide what to wear tonight. Oh right, that sweater's at the cleaners. What about the blue one? Breathe, breathe. Say the mantra. I really have to pee.

After a week, I return to the realm of the White Coats to have blood drawn. Keith Agre's back; and when he asks how I'm feeling, I blabber on about the lingering effects of altitude sickness, and the "die-off" from detoxing (I've been on a steady diet of green drinks mixed with apples and beets from my local health food store). "And, I've been meditating," I add.

Keith watches me with a bland expression that must be very difficult to sustain and says evenly, "I should have test results tomorrow afternoon. I'll call you."

Tomorrow comes with the lab results: no change. My liver is still out of whack, so more tests, PET scan, CT scan. Keith's voice grows serious. "We'll probably need to do a biopsy."

Biopsy. That word. Biopsy followed by a phone call, followed by a doctor's appointment, followed by more chemo.

This would be the time for my body's own ability to heal to kick in, but I don't seem to possess the trigger. My symptoms have not subsided; if anything, they've gotten worse. I'm still sleeping ten hours a night and still waking up tired. Meditation goes badly. If only I could master it again, the anxiety would dissipate. The flame of butterflies would quietly fold their wings again.

As determined as I am, I cannot sit still. My body feels like an exposed nerve, a giant toothache from the top of my head to the bottom of my toes.

I'm terrified.

With the leaves falling and the deer

fattened, it is time to hunt. Since the fields

have been reaped, hunters can easily

see fox and the animals which have come

out to glean. The men ride over

the stubble of reaped grain fields pursuing

their prey by the light of the moon. They

ride till the horses' hooves begin to bleed.

Lakota Sioux

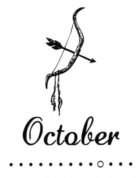

October

· · · · · · · · · · · ◦ · · ·

THE HUNTER'S MOON

I love synchronicity. Synchronicity assures me that everything is still working. The Old Geezer is right up there on his
cloudbank stopping the rain for me. Early in the morning, Carol
Moss calls to say she's got a healer staying at her house in Malibu,
a Croatian currently living in Germany who's a friend of her son-
in-law, Matthias.

Carol has already had a treatment with him for the bronchitis
that's had her down for days. The symptoms disappeared.

"Overnight! He's amazing," she says. "Get right down here!"

Without a second's hesitation, without a change of clothes or
a dab of make-up, I jump in the car.

Carol's daughter, Diane, greets me at the door. Carol is
upstairs resting after her session. We go into the glass-enclosed
lanai overlooking the beach where a massage table's been set
up; and Diane introduces me to Paulo. He is tall and wide-
shouldered with high cheekbones and a sweeping brow. His
gray-brown hair is pulled back in a long pony tail. He is dressed
in a striped soccer shirt and khaki pants and looks astonishingly

like a Native American.

"Paulo Klikovic," he says with a broad smile as he takes my hand. I smile back. He looks strangely familiar. Could I have met him before? Not likely. Strains of a flute, Native American sounds, come from a CD player. German-born Matthias will come in after the session and translate for Paulo.

I lie on my back, close my eyes and listen to the sounds of the surf outside the window. I feel Paulo's heat-lamp hands moving above me, scanning my body, pausing in places, concentrating the heat on trouble spots where energy might be blocked. This is the Native American way of getting energy flowing, breaking up any blockages with the heat of hands. I cannot imagine where Paulo has learned this technique, but I can't ask him. Paulo does not speak a word of English.

Instead, I just allow the sacred healing to flow through me. My breath rises and falls with the sighing of the surf. Each wave is a breath—inhale, exhale, inhale, exhale. I am pure essence. I am the sea, I am the sun, I am the wind and the earth. I am the clear blue sky that fills my mind and stretches on into eternity.

After what might have been an hour, maybe two, I hear his voice. "Hello," he says.

I force my eyes open.

Paulo stands over me, smiling. His blue eyes are soft and kind, and once again I am reminded of someone.

It takes me a while, but finally, very slowly, I stand and re-inhabit my body. It is as if a soft wind has blown through me, taking with it every ache and pain. I can't believe it. Can this possibly last?

"Thank you," I murmur. "Danka." The words are hardly adequate for what has just happened.

A movement from beyond the glass causes me to turn. A stone's throw from the shore there is a pod of dolphins, 20 or more, their great blue-gray bodies smooth as marble glistening in the sunlight. They are doing a spectacular dance, bursting up and out of the water, spewing a circle of white foam and then rolling back into a graceful dive. Paulo sees it, too. We watch, awed.

"Look!" I call out to the others. "Come see this!"

Diane and Matthias rush in from the living room. We stand watching in silence until the dolphins disappear from sight. It is as fine a ceremony as I have ever seen anywhere in the world. They appeared as if summoned by the energy Paulo created in that room, much the way animals in the forest appear to be witnesses, perhaps to Native American rites.

Matthias and Paulo begin to talk. Matthias translates for me. "Paulo says there is nothing really wrong with your liver, just some inflammation that has nothing to do with cancer. Anyway, he's fixed it."

That night I sleep the sleep of angels and wake refreshed and renewed without a trace of pain anywhere in my body. My mind is still a cloudless clear blue sky.

I call Agre and ask if we can do one more blood test before we do any further investigations. "I've been to see this healer," I explain, "and I know there's nothing wrong with my liver now."

I can practically hear Keith's eyes rolling back in his head, but he agrees, grudgingly, to repeat the blood test again. Two days later, the report comes back: liver enzymes are back to normal.

I know all the arguments. I've even written about them: the placebo effect, the normal self-correcting, self-limiting of a passing condition. This was none of these. This was a true healing.

It isn't until days later that I realize why Paulo looked familiar. He is the healer who came to me in my fevered dream months before.

I want more. I want every last one of those undetectable cells hiding inside me neutralized, blown away, blasted. Only a powerful healer can do this by flooding the body with energy and stimulating the body's own immune system.

After Paulo leaves to return home to Germany, I go on the hunt for other healers within driving distance. My blood counts are still way too low to travel. I'm told one sneeze from someone anywhere on the plane could land me in the hospital.

I enter "Energy healers + California" in a search engine and get an astounding 1,320,000 hits, one on every street corner it seems. I scroll through the pages. They all claim to heal everything from tennis elbow to cancer, and they can do it over the phone! They post photographs of themselves. The women all look like failed actresses turned real estate agents and have cute names that end in "i." The men look like used car salesmen. This is worrisome to me. When I wrote about healers, I had to travel all over the world, climb mountains, ride buses along dusty backroads, duck into mud huts. Now, ten years later, it seems I can just pick up the phone and give my credit card number and presto! Arthritis, backache, migraine, carpal tunnel, and sure, cancer, gone for good.

I'm discouraged. Much as I believe in energy healing, buying all of the snake-oil sales pitches would be stretching my belief well beyond the breaking point. I've met true healers and many self-appointed, self-deluded fake ones. You can spot the difference a mile away: first in the eyes where their gift shines through, warm and bright, like candleglow, and then in the hands, which will be open and expressive in a gesture of giving. A true healer will charge very little and be willing to take less, or no money at all if a person can't pay. Any offering is accepted humbly and gratefully. I have yet to meet a true healer who will take credit for his or her gift. It is a gift given by God or the Creator, they believe, and it is to be shared generously and lovingly with those in need. Then, there are the so-called healers, like the one the man in the plane spoke of who charge huge sums of money and, if questioned, will ask you what you think your life is worth. I'm thinking I will have to wait until I am able to travel to Brazil again.

· · · · · · · · · · · ·

But then, another synchronistic moment! I am walking down the street in the nearby village of Larchmont, when I spot a face that seems familiar, yet so far out of context it takes me until I am perhaps 20 feet away before I place it. Bebeto! I turn to him at the same moment he turns back to get a second look at me. We laugh, delighted, and hug.

I had met Bebeto in Brazil at the Spiritist Center Frei Luiz in Japarepaquá outside Rio, where he volunteered as an assistant to the healers and a guide and translator for English-speaking visitors. I had tagged along with other visitors—doctors and scientists from England and Germany—on a fact-finding mission through South America to explore other cultures' knowledge of healing. Bebeto and I became friends while I was in Brazil, meeting often for dinner in one of his favorite off-the-beaten-track cafes in Rio and talking late into the night.

Bebeto, a fine-looking, soft-spoken man in his 50s, began life in the favelas. His teen years were marked with violence and crime until he discovered books and, soon after, his gift of healing. He learned English from the movies that he snuck into almost daily.

Over dinner one night in Rio with a few of his friends, one of them told me Bebeto had brought his grandmother back from death. She had suffered a heart attack while she was in a hospital. The doctor, having pronounced her dead, left the room; but Bebeto stayed. He stood over his grandmother, praying and holding his hands above her chest until she began to breathe again. Bebeto then had her transferred to the Spiritist Center's elders' home where he enlisted as a volunteer. He met a professor there, also a volunteer, who helped him get a scholarship to the University of Rio, where he studied filmmaking. Recently, Bebeto completed a documentary on Spiritism that was well received at several festivals.

Spiritism (not to be confused with spiritualism, popular in America in the 1800s), Bebeto explained on that first tour of the campus, is not a religion but a philosophical doctrine that incorporates religion, science and philosophy and is based on the belief in reincarnation and the possibility of communication between the living and the spirit world.

Spread across several hundred acres of what was once a sugarcane plantation, the center, Frei Luis, was the most revolutionary community I had ever seen—a utopia. There were perhaps a dozen buildings on the campus: an orphanage for abandoned children, a school, a home for the elderly, a homeopathic clinic, a huge lecture hall, and classrooms for both school age kids and adults, all built with donations.

The hospital, where energy healings occur as well as "spiritual" operations, treats more than 3,000 people two times a week, all free of charge. From what I could see, it was the seedbed of a radical social movement as well.

I was fascinated to learn that the movement draws members of the Brazilian upper-middle class: doctors, lawyers, journalists and university professors. In fact, 37% of Spiritists hold a university degree, whereas the national average of university educated Brazilians is a shocking two percent.

One day at lunch, I told Bebeto I was thinking of renting a small apartment in Rio for a few months to work on my novel.

He frowned. "I wouldn't do that," he said.

"Really? Why not?"

"You are going to need to be near your family. Some big changes are coming."

"Like what?" I asked, alarmed. "You mean like war? Another terrorist attack?"

"No," he said, his face serious. "In you."

"What do you mean?"

"You are about to experience a big shift in your life. You might lose your way for a while, but when you find it again, you will be"—he searched for the word—"*transportada*."

When I got back to the hotel, I looked up the word *transportada* in my pocket-size dictionary: transported. I still couldn't figure out what he meant. Transported where? Not to the spirit world, I hoped.

We had exchanged phone numbers. He said he planned to be in Los Angeles working on a project for a few months and promised to call me. Here he is, walking along Larchmont.

We duck into a corner café. Over coffee, I tell him about my diagnosis and ask him whether he remembers his warning. "Was this what you meant by *transportada*? Transported? Did you get the feeling then I was going to die?"

"No, no," he says reassuringly. "Not then, not now. What I meant was you were going to be transported to another level of consciousness in *this* life. Your illness has already woken you; you have a chance now to raise your frequency. Understand?"

I didn't exactly. I agree I've woken up to many things--to the preciousness of life, to the love of family and friends; but, I didn't get what he meant about frequency.

"The higher one's frequency, the more one is able to receive healing, not only on the physical level, but the spiritual level as well. To raise one's frequency is to ascend in awareness."

"How does one do that?" I ask. "Raise one's frequency?"

"With your excellent mind," he replies.

"I try, I really do—"

"Not your *head* mind," he says. "Your *heart* mind. But first you have to clean house. All of it—body, mind and spirit. Clean out the toxins in your body, release old resentments. Re*lease*, not forgive."

Seeing my quizzical look, he says, "Forgiving is for saints.

And meditate. Meditation is very important. Meditation creates a space for the healer's energy to penetrate. Healers need a clear vessel. You can't meditate using your head mind."

I nod. The blue sky mind, the Buddhists call it.

He reaches across the table and takes my hand. Closing his eyes, he says quietly, "You still have anxiety, don't you? What do you fear? Something more than dying, isn't it?"

Tears sting my eyes, I can't speak.

"Losing the life you know? This?" He waves his hand, gesturing to the other tables filled with people drinking coffee and chatting, some working on their laptops, and outside, people strolling down the street talking on cellphones, couples hand in hand, children in strollers, dogs on leashes.

I nod again, trying to smile, but I am unable to control my quivering lips.

"Sandy," Bebeto says in a voice so tender that the tears finally spill down my face. "You will be all right."

"This—this thing is finished with me now?" I ask.

Bebeto hesitates, feels my hand with both of his. "Almost. You might hit another bump in the road."

My eyes widen.

"No, no," he says. "A small one. Not to worry. Just do your work. Work is your passion, and your passion is what keeps you vital. Are you meditating?"

"Not enough."

"You must, otherwise your mind will drive you right back into fear. Fear weakens. It destroys the whole immune system."

I promise him I will do as he says. I am on a mission now. I decide I will meditate in earnest, religiously, 20 minutes in the morning, 20 minutes in the evening. After many failed attempts in which I almost pack it in, convinced I'm just not strong enough to control that wild horse of my mind, I begin to last first five minutes then ten, and after a week of sitting in the same place at the same time, I notice I've gone 20 minutes. The wild horse is at last content to stand in the sun and nibble grass while I focus my attention on the movement of air around my nostrils.

For the rest of this Hunters Moon, I stay on hunt for healers. I'm no longer a journalist now, no longer the curious observer. I am a participant in an experiment that will directly affect the outcome of my life or my death.

Incredibly, they begin to turn up. A friend I haven't seen in months calls to tell me about a Japanese acupuncturist, herbalist and energy healer who runs a clinic in New York. He happens to be in L.A., she tells me, staying at a Ramada Inn not far from me. She gives me his name and cellphone number.

I call to make an appointment to see him. Ken Kobayashi has heard about me, he says.

"Oh yes, Sandy!" he sings out. "I want to help you, I know I can help you! Come today to my hotel, I have office in my room." I'm having a hard time understanding his heavily accented English, but his laugh is infectious.

At the door of his makeshift office, he greets me with both hands, bowing slightly and smiling a Buddha-like smile.

"Come in, come in," he says excitedly, and asks me to have a seat over by the window. "We talk first," he says, and sits in a chair facing me. Ken is a small happy man, who chats nonstop about his ancestors, about chi and herbs. "No stress!" he exclaims. "Stress no good for cancer."

He has set up his hotel room as a full-service healing facility, complete with rows of bottles of herbs and tinctures, acupuncture needles, antiseptic, and cotton, all arrayed on top of the chest of drawers with military precision. I guessed him to be in his 30s, but I later learn that Ken is more than twice that.

"My family are healers for 350 years," he says. "Cancer, no problem. We find the disharmonies and correct them."

He reaches for my left hand; and for several minutes he reads my pulses, concentrating deeply, first on my wrist, then on other points along my arms. Then without my having told him, Ken tells me exactly where the problem was.

"Kidney, strong yang deficiency," he says. "Emotion of fear." He turns my hands over and examines my nails. "Yes, yes, yes, kidney. Cancer is gone now. We make sure now it doesn't come back, all right?"

On the bed there is a clean towel neatly spread out, and a folded one for the head. "You don't mind I give you acupuncture treatment?" he asks. "My needles very fine, do not hurt at all. You just relax, okay?"

It takes about an hour. I have had acupuncture before, but it always hurt, especially when they twist the needle and push it deeper into the skin. Ken's needles are magic. I drift off on a cloud of lotus petals to a land of tea ceremonies and Buddhist temples. As I leave, Ken gives me three brown paper bags containing foul-smelling herbs which he tells me to cook for 45 minutes and drink. I don't wish to hurt his feelings, but I politely decline.

I remember those herbs from years before when I tried them. It took months to get the smell out of the house, and drinking the stuff made me gag.

The next day, Ken comes to my house to check out the Feng Shui. He walks from room to room, opening kitchen cabinets, clothes closets and drawers (to my horror). Then, using Bebeto's very same words, he tells me that I must *clean house*. Literally. Get rid of all old things: clothes, objects, books, magazines. Too much clutter, he says to me, a person who thrives on clutter.

"And you must rearrange the furniture," he says. "Buddha statue goes there in the corner in front of the window." He points to the spirit house, an intricately carved miniature temple from Indonesia that sits on the top of the bookcase in my living room next to an antique wooden statue of Saint Francis from Mexico. "All spiritual things go there, facing your house."

Then, walking into my office, standing with his hands on his hips, he stares at the wall of books, the stacks of papers and, behind mirrored sliding doors, shelves containing printer, fax, modem and router and miles and miles of tangled cables and wires.

He shakes his head and says, "Do not work in this room." Instead, he tells me to work in the living room. "There." He points to the couch, which is in fact my favorite place to write, feet propped up, notebook or laptop on my lap, slumped into the worst possible position for my spine, as every chiropractor I've ever been to has told me. "I want to show you something."

He reaches into his pocket and pulls out a bobby pin. "I always have this with me," he explains. He bends over my foot and removes my shoe and pokes the side of my big toe with the bobby pin. I almost jump through the ceiling. Electricity shoots up my leg all the way into my stomach. "This is the kidney meridian," he explains.

I shake my head. Think I'll call my next book *The Japanese Healer with the Bobby Pin*.

I am doubtful about the Feng Shui, though. Rearranging the living room is a daunting prospect, one that I'm not convinced I need to do. I could move the Buddha, the spirit house and the St. Francis statue; but here in earthquake country we bolt our bookcases as well as our mirrors and heavy paintings to the wall.

. . . .

I read in the paper that Michael Mohoric, a Qigong healer from Orange County, is giving a talk at the Bodhi Tree, a wonderful bookstore in West Hollywood. Michael is a tall, strapping, All-American type, who six years ago overcame a spinal cord injury that threatened to turn him into a quadriplegic. With the help of the Tibetan master who first introduced Qigong to the United States, Michael regained the use of his legs and within a few months, his entire body. A year later he was healing others, and he found he could send his energy from anywhere.

"Time and space became the predominant thing in my awareness," he says. "Space was alive, vibrating, and extended everywhere. There really is no separation. It doesn't make any difference if I am sending energy to someone in the same room or to someone on the other side of the world. Everything is a part of consciousness."

Distance healing is a subject that both fascinates and disturbs me. I have come across it before and wrote about it. In my book on healers, I profiled Howard Wills, a man from North Carolina, who did distance healing. I couldn't quite believe it then, even when he healed a raging sore throat I had woken up with that morning, *over the phone.* I was in New Mexico for the birth of my grandson. Anthony had driven Melanie to the hospital during the night. I didn't dare stay, not with a sore throat, so I packed to leave. I was on hold with the airline when the phone buzzed, signaling I had another call. It was Howard Wills in North Carolina returning a call I had placed to him the day before. I said I'd have to call him back as I was trying to get a flight home because I'd come down with a sore throat.

"Hold on there, darlin'," he drawled. "Get off the phone with the airline and let's see if we can fix that for you." Fix it he did. Startlingly, within five minutes the sore throat had disappeared. It did not come back that day or the next or the day after that.

What happened? Somehow Howard was able to trigger my body's own immune system to subdue the inflammation and the infection that caused it. I was able to stay and welcome my new baby grandson into the family. As with so many unexplained and unfathomable events I experienced during the two years I spent researching healers and healing, I kept a corner of my (thinking) mind reserved for doubt, journalistic doubt. I didn't want to go tumbling down the wrong rabbit hole and drag my readers down there with me. And yet, I told myself, yet... Here I am, sore throat gone, holding baby AJ in my arms.

The best explanation I got about distance healing came from a British physicist I met when I was in Abadiania in Brazil. He was one of the doctors and scientists there to observe the work of John of God. "Healing," the physicist explained, "is just the transfer of energy. Much of our everyday energy is transferred to us over great distances, whether wired or wireless. Satellite dishes for example, radio waves, the cellphone and wired landline all have to do with energy. Energy travels faster than the speed of light through time and space." He quoted Albert Einstein's explanation of the radio: "'You see, a wire telegraph is a kind of a very, very long cat. You pull his tail in New York and his head is meowing in Los Angeles. Do you understand this? Radio operates exactly the same way: you send signals here, they receive them there. The only difference is that there is no cat.' The same principle holds true for energy." Einstein is said to have come up with the theory of relativity while imagining himself riding on a ray of light. An indication perhaps that he was capable of thinking with both his mind and his heart at the same time.

· · · · · · · · · · · ·

During this moon of the hunter I have begun to assemble my team of healers. I am in familiar terrain now; all I have to do is to keep my frequencies raised and my heart-mind open, and my "houses" clean.

We are thankful to good herbs

for healing us when we are sick.

And for all the animals for keeping

our precious forests clean;

for the trees that shade us and keep

us warm; and for all the birds in

the world for singing their

beautiful songs.

Cherokee Children's Morning Song

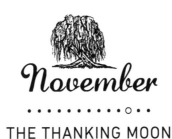

November

· · · · · · · · · · ○ · ·

THE THANKING MOON

It is a rite of passage to have one's child take over the family ritual of holiday dinners. I have to admit that Billy, together with HJ, is much better at it than I ever was. Their way of entertaining is more creative; they're always experimenting with new dishes and newly discovered wines.

This Thanksgiving, Billy is doing two huge turkeys. One is roasted the traditional way; the other is deep fried in a 40-quart pot attached to a propane gas-tank outdoors behind the kitchen. We are 24 at table, another six at a kiddies table. I make my johnnycakes.

None of the other sibs is here. They are each in their own homes with their own families, but we spoke on the phone in the morning. I had gotten up early, made tea, and called first Mark in New Hampshire, which is three hours later. Sally and Dick and Debbie were on the East coast too. Anthony in New Mexico was only an hour later. Last came Wendy in Northern California.

"I have so much to be thankful for," I said. I want to say more. I want to tell them how humbled I am by their generosity of spirit, and how very proud I am of the people each of them has become.

"I am so very grateful for you," is all I could manage without my voice going on me and breaking my own rule of banning poignancy while still in the Land of Cancer.

It's a chilly morning. I open a closet to get a sweater and see the dozen or so framed photographs still stacked there from the time I moved in that I somehow never got around to hanging. Bill had studied photography with famed photographer Bruce Davidson; consequently, we are a very well-archived family: fat-cheeked, smiling babies, then as toddlers at the beach, then as teenagers in goggles and caps streaking down a ski slope. Here's Anthony holding up the ten-pound grouper he had just caught and another of all six gathered around a table at Mark's twelfth birthday party.

As I lay the photographs out on the floor, positioning them the way I want them on the wall, scenes come alive for me. I stop a moment and let them play on my mind's screen, slowing the film down when I come upon a scene that I want to linger on, or some important detail I must not forget.

We're in Paris. I am standing in front of a bateau mouche, Notre Dame rising in the background. We had dinner that night at Lasserre and walked back to our hotel. I wanted to go hear music afterwards, but Bill, a recovering alcoholic, (never say recovered, he taught me) didn't like to go to clubs. I argued that one did not have to drink to listen to music. He grew cold and silent as he often would, maddeningly, putting an end to further discussion. I was furious. "Please don't do this. Not in *Paris* for god's sake!" The next morning, by way of apology, Bill agreed to go with me to Givenchy (we had a letter of introduction), where I bought a pink silk sheath that fit perfectly, except for the length. Charming, elegant Hubert de Givenchy told me that Audrey Hepburn had this dress in a few colors.

I laughed. "Then clearly Miss Hepburn is a woman of excellent taste," I said. Hubert had it ready for me later that day.

What else do I remember from that trip? I concentrate on calling up even the smallest snippets of memory, and a Joseph Conrad quotation comes to mind: "In plucking the fruit of memory one runs the risk of spoiling its bloom." No, it is Thanksgiving, a day to try to come to terms with those moments that were turning points in my life, while I still can, and to sort them out. I pluck on, savoring each fruit.

We're at Versailles standing in the garden where a daffy Englishwoman, who reminded us of Margaret Rutherford, offered to take our picture but couldn't find the viewfinder and took a picture of the bottom half of a rosebush instead. Bill had taken a picture of the gigantic peaches that were put in our room every day that he couldn't stop eating, at least not until he was gripped by stomach cramps in the middle of the night. Even then he blamed it on the oysters we'd had at dinner.

Where did we go next? Oh yes, I must not forget that wonderful drive from Paris to the South. We stopped along the way for gas and discovered, much to our surprise, five or six tables set up beneath umbrellas behind the gas station. We took seats, and the woman whose husband pumped the gas asked if we were hungry. Carrying a squirming baby on her hip, she brought us a carafe of wine. We watched chickens pecking at the grass, two dogs chasing each other, and a small goat roaming free. When our lunch, the best in all of France, we said (cold roast chicken, white asparagus, endive salad and cheese and fabulous wine) was ready, the woman handed me the baby so she could serve it to us.

I come across pictures of other Thanksgivings. Here's the year we piled the kids, all six, into the Beechcraft and flew to Bimini and had conch fritters and pompano instead of turkey. Here's another in Sun Valley to ski, or maybe that was Christmas; and, we mailed our gifts ahead to be placed under the tree that was set up for us.

The next Christmas we spent at our farm in Connecticut, the last place Bill and I lived together. It's an idyllic place of rolling green pastures in spring and summer; beautiful in autumn too, when the trees burst into color and the sunsets turn the sky deep red.

That winter an ice storm hit Connecticut. Power lines were encased in ice and our house went dark. The storm hit just about the time our marriage began to freeze. Outside, the world turned to crystal, silent, except for the occasional loud crack of a frozen branch breaking loose and hitting the ground. Inside, small disagreements turned into silences and doors were slammed shut. Our king-size bed became the loneliest place on earth with acres of empty space spread out between our turned backs.

The phone rang, startling me out of my reverie. Realizing it had been ringing off the hook, I ran to grab it. It was Billy, calling to tell me that we had six last minute additions to dinner and asking me if I would come over sooner to get started on the johnnycakes. "Sure," I said. I started to stack the photographs to put them back in the closet. What was I doing anyway, letting myself get drawn down a memory lane that was strewn with land mines? Well, unhealed wounds are land mines too, I decide. They can poison the environment that allows cancer to flourish, so johnnycakes will have to wait.

What happened to our marriage? The ice storm passed, and the ice on the trees and power lines finally thawed. Our marriage remained frozen at the center.

That spring we went to a black tie dinner in New York. I wore the pink silk Givenchy. There are two kinds of flirting. There's the kind that's an amusing, harmless game much like an after-dinner game of bridge. Then there's the kind that prompts a phone call the next day. Oh, how I want to re-shoot that scene.

Years later, I tried once to tell Bill how I regretted that affair. We had just come from his doctor's, and we were sitting side by side in a restaurant. The waiter interrupted, and I thought the moment had passed. I reached into my bag and showed him the new pen I'd just bought. He took it out of my hand and on a cocktail napkin wrote the words, *I love you.* I came across that napkin sometime later. It was stuck between some unframed photographs in a file marked "Personal," and I cried.

It occurs to me that this might not be what Bebeto meant by cleaning house; this is regret, plain bitter-tasting regret. I feel no sense of release, just the sting of wounds reopened.

· · · · · · · · · · · ·

Now, at Billy's and HJ's Thanksgiving dinner, I go outside to observe the ceremonial dunking of the bird into boiling oil.

Billy explains that he had injected the turkey with seasonings and marinated it overnight. Without looking at me, he asks, "So I gather your liver enzymes are back to normal?"

"Oh yes," I reply. "It was just some sort of inflammation that ran its course." I pause a beat. "Apparently."

I do not mention my healing session with Paulo. In fact, I haven't told anyone in the family about it. This is strange, because the girls are quite interested in natural ways of healing. Maybe my reticence has to do with a thought that has been marinating in my mind ever since the last liver test.

I'm still not a hundred percent decided, but I don't think I want to continue these routine tests, the PET/CT scans, the blood work, and most of all the twice-yearly cystoscopy that's part of the post-chemo protocol—at least not as long as I'm symptom free. I don't presume to know what I would do if, for instance, I started peeing buckets of blood again. Barring that scary turn of events, I'm beginning to feel I'm safer with alternative doctors and healers and with my body's ability to absorb enough of their energy to heal itself. This is at least what I am considering.

Billy is very much his father's son. If Bill were here, he would strenuously object to the decision forming in my mind and get Billy and the rest of the family to gang up on me. He did just that 15 years ago, when I wanted to choose the alternative route to deal with breast cancer. Although we were divorced by that time, Bill called me on the phone. "You couldn't be more mistaken," he said sternly. "You must not do that." Just as if we were still married. A mutual friend of ours, who lived near Bill's beach house, called me to say that Bill had knocked on her door late at night. He was in tears. She said he told her what was going on with me and how worried he was that I might refuse traditional treatment. He begged her to call me and try to talk some sense into me.

A week later in Los Angeles over lunch with Billy, I told him that I really believed in alternative medicine over allopathic treatment and that I wanted to go that route. I watched my son's eyes grow moist.

"And if that doesn't work," he asked, "what then? What about me?"

That did it. My son's tears would probably break my resolve again. I still wonder whether Bill had prompted Billy to say that to me.

I am hypnotized by the bird boiling away in the caldron. *Round about the caldron go; In the poison'd entrails throw… Double double toil and trouble…*

"Mom, stand back! It might splatter."

Wait a minute. Does it really have to be an either or question? Why the duality? Why can't it be either and both? If chemo is used sparingly and followed up by various methods of cleansing and detoxing and rebuilding the immune system along with some very deep changes in the psyche to trigger the body's own capacity to complete the healing process, why not? Maybe in fact, this is what I am proving with my own recovery. Maybe it's time for Humpty Dumpty to hop down off the wall. That wall might be imaginary.

When Father sun has traveled

south to his home to rest before he

starts back on his journey north.

Then, once again there will be warmth

and light upon the land.

Abenaki

December

• • • • • • • • • • • ○ •

THE TURNING MOON

It's Christmas time; the sky is blue, and the weather balmy. I put all questions of tests and treatments out of my mind and rejoice. I rejoice as I do my Christmas shopping: Tommy Bahama shirt for Anthony, book on tape for Mark, sweater for Billy (otherwise known as the dreaded Christmas sweater), cookbook for HJ, wine for Sally and Dick, baskets of cookies and teas for Wendy and Deb, and a swing through Toys R Us for the little boys. Anthony will advise me on gifts for AJ and Alec.

I rejoice as I buy a tabletop tree of fragrant rosemary to place on my coffee table and decorate it with tiny lights and ornaments. I curl up on the couch beside it and write my cards. I even rejoice as I weave my way through holiday traffic, humming along with the incessant, mindless holiday music on the radio. When I find a parking spot right away I feel that this world is my creation and I am all powerful in it. Just this, I say quietly. This is all I need. *Just this.*

I buy some new clothes—a pair of shoes, a handbag. I get my hair (!) done. I go to dinners and cocktail parties; and over lunch

I exchange gifts with friends, each painstakingly wrapped with carefully worded notes tied to the ribbon.

Alex gives me yet another beautiful painting she found on this year's trip to Brazil, a beach scene in the naïve style. My novel's fictional Peter had suddenly begun to paint in this style after the New Year's Eve beach ceremony.

Masha has brought a small, colorful rug back from whatever obscure country she's just been to—one of the Stans, I think. There's a book about Paris from Terry and Jan. A certificate for a massage comes from Billy and HJ, wine from Dick and Sally, and a sweater from Wendy with a card addressed to Beloved Wick. Packages fly back and forth across the country. Some--mystery packages with no return addresses or names I recognize—I've stacked in a corner of the living room, to be opened Christmas morning before I go over to Billy and HJ's. Each morning, emails pop up on my laptop from friends I haven't heard from in ages with family photographs attached.

Betty Fussell blows into town. She's researching her new book on the history of beef in America and is headed for a cattle ranch outside Santa Barbara. I'll go with her; we can have dinner at the Hitching Post, the restaurant featured in the movie "Sideways". I've had some joint pains—left knee and lower back—nothing terrible, probably just toxins working their way out of my body. I won't report it; this is nothing I can't live with.

Another day an old friend from New York calls to say she's in town. We have lunch at my neighborhood Italian restaurant and polish off a bottle of wine and talk our heads off.

The phone is ringing as I walk into my apartment. A man's

voice sounding vaguely familiar asks to speak to me. It's Jack, an old love, more than an old love, actually. He's someone I married briefly after a whirlwind summer romance in Montauk. The marriage was sweet but didn't last. We had it annulled a few months later by mutual agreement. He's calling to say he's planning to be in L.A. in a few weeks and asks if I would like to have dinner. I smile at the idea.

My awful odyssey into the Land of the Ill has come to an end. I understand why it came and heard what it was it had to tell me, now it's gone. I can fill my life with ordinary normal, wondrous activities.

I cancel my December appointments with Keith Agre and Quinn and send them both Christmas cards instead. I decide to cancel my PET/CT scans too. I'm much too busy living my life in this holiday season. If anything is going on in my back or joints, I don't want to hear about it. Not now, not at Christmas, maybe not ever. This last thought stops me. Do I mean that? Am I really prepared now to take full responsibility for my own health and healing and to what extent? To the extent of Christmas, anyway, I decide and put it out of my mind. Was Christmas always this wonderful? Funny how in all these years I hadn't noticed.

Only one thing is missing, and it's really missing. I wake up one morning longing for a puppy. A *puppy*. Dare I? It's one thing to leave grown children with families of their own behind. That's in the natural order of things. In return for the unconditional love and loyalty, the adoring gaze, the frantic leaping and twirling and wagging that greets us every time we walk in the door, we agree to be there for a dog; it's a sacred trust.

A "familiar" is what witches called them, a cat, dog, snake, frog, bird or any creature whose job it was to assist them with their magic. Native Americans called upon them in shamanistic rites and named them power animals. A familiar heals too. When I was undergoing treatment for breast cancer, my Shar Pei, Chin Chin, used to lie tight against me, leaving me only to quickly eat or use the doggie door and then gently, softly jump back up onto the bed or couch where I was resting. Tashi Delek, my Maltese who long before Paris Hilton made a dog an silly accessory, road around in my shoulder bag to restaurants, movie theatres, and even airplanes (before 9/11). He even walked down the aisle with me at Billy's and HJ's wedding.

The Dalai Lama was right: too much attachment. Pets die and leave you broken-hearted. Worse though by far is for us to die and leave them homeless and without their person.

I call Alex. She's had a couple of bouts with cancer herself and she has two cats.

"What do you think?" I ask after I've told her what's on my mind.

"Of course!" she practically shouts. "You have to have a puppy."

Alex once worked in veterinary clinics and knows her way around the animal kingdom. I had already found a breeder of Maltese 30 miles away.

"Will you come with me?" I ask.

"In a flash."

We drive out to a place outside Pasadena that has Maltese puppies. They are adorable, they are delightful. The problem is they aren't Tashi.

Alex picks up a sweet little ten-week-old female and hands her to me. "What about this one?"

I take her into my arms and smile. "Cute," I admit, "but not Tashi."

They are all cute, and none of them is Tashi. I am about to give up and leave, when suddenly a jet black ball of fluff comes streaking into the room and pounces on a large ball. She rolls it and chases it, trying to get her mouth around it. When she realizes she can't, she pounces on it again, this time hard enough to make it bounce in the air then chases it again. She will not give up. The little Maltese pups don't move a hair; they just watch.

"What is that?" I ask the kennel owner.

"A Brussels Griffon. Unusual color, they're generally various shades of brown, like the one in the movie, "As Good As It Gets" with Jack Nicholson."

Of course. Same personality, same expression, same monkey face. After a moment the little black dynamo runs to me and looks up at me with huge eyes, tail wagging furiously, and dares me to say no. This one exudes a fierce determination to love life, to live. I scoop her up and name her Charley (my nickname for Hanuman the Hindu monkey god). Mark flies in, and we go shopping for Charley gear—bed, collar and leash, wee-wee pads, toys, bones, food, dishes, crate.

"You're kidding," one writer friend says. "How do you expect to get any work done with a new puppy around barking and peeing on the rugs and chewing up the house?"

"No problem," I say with great bravado. "I've done it before."

The housebreaking is a snap. Charley is incredibly smart, but she's a tornado! She has enough energy to power Hoover Dam and light up all of Las Vegas and half of Los Angeles. It isn't a problem. I laugh as she bounces around with her toys. I get in extra walks and try to get her not to tug and twirl and buck at the end of the leash like some mad, wild pony. She does, however, chew the cord to my laptop.

I had been keeping a careful journal about my travels into the Land of Cancer; and following my epiphany at the turkey caldron, I was now deep into fresh research. I had come across the work of a German physician, Dr. Ryke Geerd Hamer, who explores the emotional causes of cancer and why it appears in a particular organ. I thought about what it means that I got hit in the kidney and bladder. Was there something, for instance, that I was pissed off about? Quite a lot, it would seem. Following that reasoning, anger weakens the kidney and makes it fertile terrain for cancer to grow. Did I have anything to be angry about? Oh yes. Got a minute?

In another book, *Cancer is Not a Disease,* the Ayurvedic practitioner, Andre Moritz, says, "He who finds purpose and meaning in the occurrence of a cancerous tumor will also find the way to cure it."

I uncovered other radical theories. Microbiologist Dr. Robert Young, who runs a clinic in Orange County, claims that "... Cancer is not a cell at all; it is a poisonous acidic liquid that has been spoiled or poisoned by metabolic or gastrointestinal acids. Cancer is a systemic acidic condition that settles at the weakest parts of the body; a tumor is the body's protective mechanism to encapsulate spoiled or poisoned cells from excess acid that has not been properly eliminated through urination, perspiration, defecation or respiration. The tumor is the body's solution to protect surrounding healthy cells and tissues." If what Dr. Young is saying is true, then the way cancer is treated with the holy trinity of modern Western medicine—chemo, radiation and surgery—would be all wrong. Dr. Tullio Simonici, an Italian oncologist, believes chemo and radiation both cause cancer later on. Of all the doctors and scientists I interviewed, he is by far the most radical. His book, *Cancer is a Fungus,* states that cancer is in fact the fungus, Candida Albicans, and responds to the simple and inexpensive treatment of sodium bicarbonate orally or by injection directly into the site of the tumor. Dr. Simonici also believes chemo and radiation are both carcinogens.

It seems then, if we were to put fifty leading doctors and cancer research scientists in a room and ask them each to explain what cancer is and how to heal it, we'd get fifty conflicting answers. So where does that leave us? Dr. Albert Schweitzer has an answer, "Each patient carries his own doctor inside him. They come to us not knowing that truth. We are at our best when we give the doctor who resides within each patient a chance to work."

I believe that. The burning question for me is, how do we find that doctor within? If we do happen to find him, how can we be sure we can trust him, that he's not a snake-oil salesman posing as a doctor?

I go back to the novel. I was facing a dilemma in that world too. I couldn't kill off the character Peter. He had become too much a part of me, but I wasn't sure how to snatch him from the gods he had angered.

That's when Charley the monkey god steps in. Suddenly my computer screen goes black. I gasp, look down and see the mangled cord. Everything's gone! Two hundred and fifty pages dispatched into the ether, vanished in a flash into the spirit world of cyberspace. In a panic I call Mark.

"Relax, it's okay," he says. "I can restore all the pages you lost." He will order me a new cord; and, then with his shamanic computer powers, he will connect his computer to mine (see, we really are all one) and bring my fictional world back to me. That will take a few days, though; meantime I am without my novel.

I am forced to turn to my notebook. Page after page is filled with notes about my diagnosis and thoughts about my healing. I begin to add other memories to see whether I can start to make some sense of it all, this cancer. I write for hours, even into the night, something I never do. I know I can only understand my experience by using my pen to excavate the truth and look at it on paper with a clear eye. It has to be in there somewhere. It has to be; it's been calling to me to all along. I have simply ignored its voice, until the monkey god pulled the plug to the computer, forcing me to turn to the pen.

My new familiar also brought me a new guide to the world of healers. One day, while in the pet store buying toys, I notice a card on the counter: "Chris' Critter Sitter, Dog Walking, Puppy Training, Day Care Services." The eponymous Chris lives five minutes from me. The store owner tells me he uses her himself. She keeps his dog in her house when he has to go away. Chris is great, he says, the best.

I call the number on the card, and Chris agrees to come by to meet me and Charley. Chris Rungé is a presence. Tall and sturdy with close-cropped snow-white hair, her face tanned from running dogs and taking care of all manner of animals—dogs, rabbits, horses at a nearby stable whose denizens also include a pig and goat and several cats. Her smile is warm and engaging. Charley leaps onto Chris' lap and kisses her the minute she sits down, as if she were a long lost best friend. As we talk, we discover that our paths have crossed many times: in Pennsylvania at the Devon Horse Show years before; in Abadiania, Brazil where she had been the year after I had gone. She also knew several of the healers that I have written about. Chris has been drawn to healing and healers all her life, just as her mother, an author and seeker, before her was. Charley is welcome to join her assortment of pups for a few hours a day, she tells me. It's a kind of pre-kindergarten for canines where they learn to get along with all manner of critter, no matter color, breed or creed.

I tell her she should run one for humans. It seems she does. One night a month, Chris leads a meeting called the Circle of Friends, based on the teachings of Bruno Groening, a famous German healer long dead but whose miraculous healings are still carried on by his many followers worldwide. She promises to invite me to the next Bruno meeting.

· · · · · · · · · · · ·

In this Turning Moon, as I look back over the past 12 moons, I see that chemo had a very definite place in my recovery. I did not have the maximum sub-lethal dose, where the oncologist brings the patient almost to the brink of death and then tries

to salvage what's left of her. I was lucky; I had a more conserva-
tive oncologist, Dr. David Quinn, who used a restrained dose to
debulk the tumor, giving my body's own natural defense mechanism a chance to take over. It also gave me time to change the
body's terrain. Starting with the mind, where awareness resides,
then moving into the heart, the seat of the soul according to some;
and, then flooding the rest of the body with healing energy into the
organs and finally to the cells themselves, who are always listening.
According to Bruce Lipton, "…each cell is an intelligent being that
can survive on its own, as scientists demonstrate when they remove
individual cells from the body and grow them in a culture…these
smart cells are imbued with intent and purpose; they actively seek
environments that support their survival while simultaneously
avoiding toxic or hostile ones. Like humans, single cells analyze
thousands of stimuli from the microenvironment they inhabit.
Through the analysis of this data, cells select appropriate behav-
ioral responses to ensure their survival."

I have come to understand that healing is both an art and a
science. Each of us in need of healing is a crucible in which that
combinatory alchemy must take place—with the mind, first and
foremost, the mind. Wendy had given me her favorite book on
Buddhism, *The Heart of Buddhist Meditation* by the great scholar,
Nyanaponika Thera. I pick it up from time to time and re-read
the words that have particular meaning for me right now: "…
human beings still bungle only with the symptoms of their malady,
remaining blind to the source of the illness." In the Buddhist
doctrine, mind is the starting point, the focal point, and the
culminating point.

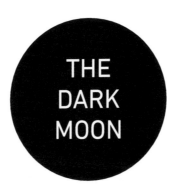

THE
DARK
MOON

A year and seven months have passed since I had my last chemo. My energy is back and so is my hair. I continue my 'quest' as Judith calls it, investigating and interviewing more healers. I fly to Montana with Chris to see Dr. Jim MacKimmie, a healer she discovered through his book, *Presence of Angels; a Healer's Life*. A former chiropractor with a thriving practice in Northern California, he had picked up and moved to the wilds of Montana where he sees people from all over the world who've heard of his miraculous healings. I see him over a period of three days and come away convinced I have met one of the most gifted healers on the planet.

I conduct interviews with my White Coats too. Both Keith Agre and David Quinn agree to sit down with me and discuss their beliefs and philosophies about medicine. Quinn grew up in Australia around aboriginals and their shamanistic ways, but he chose the opposite path of scientific exploration. He chose oncology, because it held the most challenge.

Although Keith Agre's office is in Beverly Hills, he is far from anyone's idea of a Beverly Hills doctor. A specialist in nephrology, his practice is mainly internal medicine. To say that he doesn't suffer fools and their vitamins gladly is a major understatement. When I first started going to him, and named all the supplements I was taking, he responded in his gravelly voice, "Congratulations, you have the most expensive urine in Los Angeles." Yet, he did suffer me, kindly and with deep compassion when I needed him most. I trusted his judgment. Because of that trust, he helped make me believe I could heal, which is the ultimate placebo.

Cell biologist Bruce Lipton explains the effect of that placebo. "We're born with doctors; we learn as children that when we're sick our parents take us to the doctor. In this developmental phase, the program is very clear. But what's interesting is we're really able to heal ourselves. And then you say, well how come we just don't always heal ourselves? And the answer is because most of us were given a program that says you don't heal yourself, the doctor heals you. I've got to tell you though; I wouldn't want to live without the medical profession. Why? Because if I'm in an accident, I don't want a chiropractor sewing me up. If I need a heart transplant, then homeopathy is not the direction I want to go. Conventional medicine works miracles in anything when it comes to trauma. It's just when you get outside the range of trauma, the effectiveness declines significantly."

I make an appointment to see Dr. Mary Hardy, a nutritionist at UCLA, who believes deeply in the necessity of profound change even beyond diet and nutrition. She outlines a diet program but reminds me that's only a part of the work that lays ahead for me. "Change, on a profoundly deep level that rewrites the trajectory of the story is what's needed, the story that brought you to this moment in time."

Body repair is needed too. I see cranial-sacro therapist Sandra Capelli for lymphatic drainage treatments to keep the lymphatic system clear.

I'd been hearing about a man I'll call Dr. Darling (you'll see why in a minute). He's a former oncologist-turned-nutritionist, who left oncology because his patients were not getting well or getting well until the next recurrence. He'd be happy to see me, he said and suggested I fax him my records ahead of time.

The moment I walked into his very plush office, he hugged me and called me Darling and made us both a cup of herbal tea. I couldn't take my eyes off his blinding Hollywood white teeth set off by his deep tan. After a bit of small talk, mostly about the sad state of medicine, he got down to the business of my records. "As it stands now, Darling, you've got about three years before you get hit again—maybe in the other kidney, maybe in your lungs or heart or God-knows-where-else, brain, maybe or bones. Thing is, we know how to stop it." Blood draining from my face, lips trembling, ears ringing so hard I could hardly hear, I tried hard to concentrate on the protocol he was laying before me: a strict macrobiotic diet, *hundreds* of vitamins and supplements (all of which he stocked) to take several times throughout the day. I don't even remember what else. I do remember the bill though: $500 not including the vitamins, which I said I'd have to think about. I left there, expiration date stamped on my forehead, and cried all the way home.

Feeling helpless now to rewrite the trajectory of my own

story, and Mark having performed a miraculous healing on my computer, I get back to work on the novel where I and I alone am the author. I spend mornings with the novel and afternoons with the journal. I know they are connected in some way, although I still don't know exactly how. Both Peter and I are on a journey that will either take us to new awareness, a renewed way of being or to our deaths.

Finally, I go and have a PET/CT scan and a set of labs. The tests all show that I am cancer-free! Agre gives me a huge smile and declares me officially in remission. He says I ought to check in with Dr. Quinn, pop the champagne bottle with him too.

I call everyone—the boys, the girls, and my close friends—to celebrate the news. I notice I have not told anyone about Dr. Darling. I comb my bangs over my forehead to hide the expiration date.

"Charley's put you in remission," Billy says.

A day or two later, I drive to Norris for what I am certain is the last time. I find a seat on one of the couches. I scan the faces, looking for the familiar ones, but see not a single person I recognize—not the spunky little girl or the screenwriter with the laptop or the teary woman with the dire predictions. Forcing myself to think positively, I decide that, like me, they are all in remission. The little girl's hair has grown in by now and she's back in school. The writer has finished his screenplay. The woman has had her last round of chemo and is out playing tennis.

I do not stop to study the faces that have replaced the others in my cohort. Since I will not be seeing them again, I do not have to get to know them. I pick up a magazine. I flip to an article on cancer.

This year one in three people will develop cancer.
One in four people will die of cancer.
Last year, in 2005, about 1.4 million new cases of
cancer were diagnosed in the United States.
More than 1,500 Americans died each day of cancer
this year.
Over 1,000,000 new cases of skin cancer will be
diagnosed this year.
Cancer is the leading cause of death among Americans
under the age of 85.

I quickly put the magazine down and pick up the latest issue of *Vogue*, which features urgently important statistics about the latest crop of designer handbags.

A nurse calls my name. I breeze into the examining room, grinning from ear to ear at Quinn, who comes in a moment later. He reels off the standard questions: How is my appetite, am I sleeping well, getting plenty of exercise, how's the writing going?

At every turn, I am happy to report, "Fine. Great."

As I lie back on the examining table, he reads my labs, nodding.

"Good. Very good," he says.

He palpates my abdomen. "Feels fine," he says. Like Agre, he believes that I am probably in remission. Ignoring the word "probably," I sit up and button my shirt as Quinn lowers his large frame into a chair and crosses his legs, ready for a chat.

"Did you ever have that kidney removed?" he asks in a

conversational tone of voice, a tone one might use to ask whether I'd seen any good movies lately or been to the new eatery that just opened down the street.

I stare at him a moment, not sure I'm hearing right. "My kidney?" I ask. "Why would I do that?" I shake my head in disbelief. "The cancer's gone."

"Right," Quinn says, drawing the word out in his Australian accent, "but we need to have another cystoscopy. Just to make sure."

I continue to stare at him. "You mean go do that whole thing—have that camera stuck up into my kidney again? No. No, thanks." I hop off the examining table and slip into my shoes. The imaginary champagne is already getting warm. "I'm totally satisfied with the call both you and Agre have made. I am in remission." I pick up my bag, take out my valet ticket. "I'll stick with that."

"No," he says, suddenly growing uncharacteristically stern. "It's absolutely necessary at this point." He walks across the room to where the paperwork is, next to the door, blocking my exit. He stands with his back to me, making notes in my chart. "I'll call Phil Yalowitz (the urologist with the dreaded mini camera) and tell him to expect your call."

I don't answer. I'm waiting for him to move out of the way.

"If you don't call and make the appointment," he jokes, trying to lighten the mood, "I'll have to put out an APB on you." Then with a brisk pat on my shoulder, he's out of the room.

I walk out through the lobby to the door in an angry daze. This wasn't supposed to happen. I came to thank Quinn and to celebrate our victory, and now he's sending me back to square one? Cursing under my breath what a fool I was to let Agre talk me into going to see Quinn, I get into my car and gun the engine and tires screeching, head home. Have another cystoscopy? No! I won't do it. I'm done with all that. Damn White Coats! What the devil does he mean—Do I still have that kidney? What would I have done with it? Donated it to Goodwill?

I take out my cellphone to call Keith Agre but remember that he's already left for a month's vacation in Japan. I call the office and ask them to try to reach him at his hotel in Tokyo. When I get home, there is a message on my voice mail that they have tried to reach Dr. Agre, but he's already left his hotel and is hiking the Japan Alps. That's great. I think I'll go take a hike somewhere too.

I try to make contact with Schweitzer's 'doctor within' for a second opinion, but all I get is a resounding, furious No that sounds suspiciously like me. So, I do nothing the next day, or the day after that. Stubbornly, I put it out of my mind. On the third day, Yalowitz's office calls to ask which day I want to come in.

"I'll give you a call next week," I say. I'd like to wait until Agre gets back from Japan and see what he thinks. Soon after, Billy calls.

"So what did Quinn have to say?" he asks. (Seems he did put out that APB.)

I decide I will go talk to Dr. Yalowitz. "Just to talk," I emphasize to Karen, the receptionist. "I'll only need a few minutes with him." Kind, avuncular Philip Yalowitz welcomes me into his office with a hug and tells me how well I look. When I sit down, he tells me he agrees with Quinn.

"To be absolutely sure the chemo's done its job," he says, "we really do need one last look." His smile is warm, reassuring. "What's the big deal?"

The big deal is that the additional probing takes me out of the realm of *It's Over* into the realm of *What If?* The situation leaves me standing at the doors of the Land of Cancer, afraid they'll swing open and I'll be shoved back in. Yet here I am, once again unable to summon the courage to say no, not when the argument to forge ahead is so damn reasonable. It's a test, for God's sake, have it and be done with it. Then, the White Coats can all agree I am in remission and leave me alone. It's almost as if I would be a bad sport not to have had the test, like walking away from the game before I've scored an easy goal. Where exactly is the courage in that?

I insist on general anesthesia. More than photographing the interiors of my bladder and kidney, they will do a "wash" at the same time for a pathology smear, similar to a pap smear. It's done in the hospital. Including recovery time from the anesthesia, it takes only a few hours. There's no reason for Billy to leave work, and Julie offers to drive me. A nurse will call her when I'm ready to leave.

On the way to the hospital we make small talk—a show we saw on TV the night before, the weather. It's already hot this early in the morning and an awful lot of traffic for this hour. What is there to say? Julie, I'm having this test but I feel I'm copping out and I feel lousy about it, is what I want to say. But compassionate and loving as Julie is, she would frantically search for words of comfort. I don't say what's on my mind. We agree it probably won't rain today.

．． ． ． ． ． ． ． ． ． ． ． ．

Two days later, the phone call comes. "Sandy, it's Phil." I know the news before he says it. I can see it. The monster has come roaring up from the depths with blood in its eyes: "Active cancer cells have been found in the kidney."

Terrorist supercells that survived the mustard gas and Agent Orange have set up camp once again, and they are poised to strike. The kidney has to go. The monster grabs me by the neck and sinks its teeth into my gut. My three years grows closer. Fear swells up inside me.

"We've set up an appointment for you with Dr. Fuchs for tomorrow at eleven."

"Who's Dr. Fuchs?" I ask.

"You know him. Gerhard Fuchs, the surgeon." He gives me the address.

So the energy healings hadn't gotten to all the cancer cells after all. Maybe I wasn't open enough or, as Bebeto said, my houses weren't clean enough to receive the healings. I am back in the belly of the beast.

It always comes back, the woman said.

Billy reminds me this was the plan from the beginning.

"Look," he says and shows me the journal he'd been keeping. "It's all right here in my notes. Don't you remember? They were going to remove the kidney first, but then when they discovered it had already metastasized, they decided on chemo. After that, when you've recovered your strength, then they were going to do the surgery. They were always going to remove the kidney."

I frown, shake my head.

"Mom," he continues, "they never expected the chemo to get it all. I can't believe you don't remember those conversations."

I do not remember, not a bit of it. How could I? My mind had taken a powder from the day of the diagnosis. My mind wanted none of this. That's how they take over here in the Land of Cancer, a kind of mind control. The minute you walk through those portals they spray you with something so your mind will take off and you won't remember anything. I have no memory, for instance, of having been in that surgeon's office back in January to discuss a kidney operation. Even when we go back now to set up the surgery, I don't remember the doctor, and I could swear I'd never been in this office before. Finally, to prove it, Billy asked the office staff to look up my previous visit. They didn't have to; they remembered the two of us well.

The surgery is scheduled in three days. I'm told it is a minimally invasive procedure, laparoscopic nephroureterectomy, in which three or four very small incisions are made that admit tools that are only a quarter to a half-inch wide and a similarly sized viewing device called a laparoscope, which is connected to a camera. The surgeon and his team will work off of the video image displayed on a television screen. The entire operation should last about four hours, Dr. Fuchs explains, and will involve a hospital stay of four or five days.

Billy drops me off at my apartment. Charley leaps into my arms and buries her monkey nose in my neck. When I try to put her down she stands on her hind legs and frantically waves her front paws at me to pick her up again. I take to my bed, Charley curled at my side, and give myself over to despair.

Two loves I have of comfort and despair, the Shakespeare sonnet goes, *Which like two spirits do suggest me still.*

I do not shower or wash my hair or dress. At night I keep the television on to fool the demons into thinking I'm not alone.

Chris has agreed to take Charley while I'm in the hospital and keep her until I'm up and around again. How will I heal without my familiar?

Have I, like Peter in my novel, angered the goddess? I suppose I have, in so many ways. Let me count the ways. I sink deeper and deeper into the swirling dark waters that cover me and pull me down.

In the distance at first, then with an insistent loud ring, I hear the phone. Startled, I look at the clock. Eleven. I grab for the phone.

"Sandy? It's Bebeto. Hope I didn't wake you, but you were coming to me so strong in my thoughts I couldn't sleep. What time is it there?"

"Eleven. No, no, you didn't wake me. I was just in the middle of drowning."

"Is something wrong?"

"Yes. It's that bump in the road you told me about. I hit it." My voice choked with tears, I tell him first about Dr. Darling to which he yells, "Boollsheet!" then about the surgery I'm facing. "Maybe the healers' energy can't reach me. Or maybe I'm not able to absorb it. Or I don't know, maybe this cancer I have can't be healed."

"Don't be silly," he says reassuringly. "You are already healed, the doctors just don't know it. You probably would be all right without the surgery, but you might not be ready yet to believe that. It's all right. This surgery will be the end of it. It is here." He pauses a moment, and I wonder if the line's been disconnected. Then he says, "This is the time of your *transportada*."

That word again. "Bebeto, how do I know it doesn't mean transported to the spirit world?"

"Your heart knows. Turn off the television and look inside your heart."

"How did you know I have the TV on?" I ask, impressed.

"I can hear it."

. . . .

In the morning I get up early and take a long hot shower and wash my hair and get dressed. I look hard at my reflection in the mirror, searching for a sign. It is not until I take Charley out for one of our last walks and feel the cool morning breeze on my face and see the red-tail hawks wheeling, spiraling upward high above the ridge that I can focus on my heart and listen for what it has to tell me. Am I strong enough in my belief that I can heal, I ask. Or am I in fact, as Bebeto said, already healed? Am I resolute enough in that possibility to cancel the surgery or at least put it off until I am sure? The breeze is still, the trees grow quiet of birdsong, and my heart refuses to speak.

It is the second August since my last chemo, nineteen months ago. Instead of the moon, it is the hot August sun that stares me in the face, demanding a sacrifice. I am a Sun Dance pledger who must sacrifice a piece of flesh—an organ for the survival of the tribe, which is my body. I try to think of the blond, blue-eyed Teutonic surgeon as the medicine man; the hospital as my sweat lodge; the operating room as my Sun Dance grounds. It's no good. I am filled with dread. It's not a piece of flesh; it's a whole damn organ, for god's sake.

Is this the sacrifice I must make to begin the true transformation both Bebeto and Mary Hardy spoke of? Because there will always be stray cells, everyone has them. I remember reading that cancer cells occur on and off constantly in a person's lifetime. The terrain—mental, emotional and physical—has to be clean enough and strong enough to overcome them. Still, the way to take out weeds, Bebeto says, is to pull them out by the roots, get at the cause of the cancer. It is the question I have been pondering from the beginning: Is the body sick because of the cancer or is it the sickness of the person that causes the cancer? *I do know this: a life and death illness is a soul journey that can only be made alone, and barefoot.*

. . . .

Children fly in again. Chris picks up Charley. I'm due to arrive at the hospital at five in the morning. Mark drives me. We go together to the admitting desk, a cubicle of endless red tape. I have noticed that from the first moment you turn yourself over to the vast hospital system, you are no longer you. You are your birthdate, your mother's maiden name, your Social Security number, your disease and any known allergies. You are page after page of signed permissions—in triplicate—to operate, to anesthetize, to resuscitate (or not), to receive clergy (or not). You know you are not you when they call you by your given name, Sandra, the one school teachers called you and now telemarketers who call at dinnertime.

When finally we get through the mountain of paperwork, we are sent to the waiting area outside the OR. I'm stunned to find my friend, Margery Nelson, already there. She had rolled out of bed at this ungodly hour, hair slightly disheveled, without make-up. For support, she says. I have never seen anyone so beautiful.

Billy appears. He warns, "Mom, if you happen to see a white light, turn around and run like hell the other way."

I give him a wry smile. I had been talking on the phone to Mellen Thomas-Benedict, a man who became famous for his near death experience that lasted 90 minutes and changed his life. After those 90 minutes in the space he describes as The Light, he became an inventor with an extraordinary knowledge of quantum physics, biology, even medicine—knowledge that has been tested by conventional scientists.

They come for me and wheel me away, far, far away.

· · · · · · · · · · · ·

Then, voices shouting. "Breathe! Sandra, breathe!" Buzzers going off, bells ringing. "Blood pressure dropping!" A voice commands me to breathe. Too much commotion. People running into the room, shouting orders, doing things to me. I didn't really want to breathe. I wasn't ready. I hadn't seen the Light yet.

I did see something else, though. I was in a place where there were all these healers—a land, a whole beautiful land of healers. I need to get back there.

Billy and Mark were begging, "Mom, breathe!"

Just a little longer and I might have learned the meaning of existence, in that beautiful place across a sea as big as the universe, where they know.

• • • • • • • • • • • •

Hours later when I open my eyes and scan the room, I cannot figure out where I am. There's a large window, blue sky. Am I back there in that place? But why this pain? The pain in my abdomen is excruciating. I turn my head and see Julie. She is sitting in a chair quietly meditating. How did she get here? I've got to see one of those healers and do something about this pain. When I open my eyes again, Julie's still there. Billy is here too, speaking to doctors. In the corner of the room is a cot. It's a huge room with a sitting area. Mark is sitting on it, holding his head in his hands. He's distressed. Oh, that's right. I'm in the hospital. They took my kidney.

When I wake up again, a doctor is speaking to me. I'm trying to follow what he's saying, something about by removing the kidney the cancer is back at Stage I. I blink hard, trying to comprehend. "…and the cancer cells were all in situ, meaning it hadn't invaded any surrounding tissue."

Another doctor is saying "…a blood transfusion… the kidney had gotten stuck to the structure surrounding it… quite a lot of blood loss…"

Mark comes and sits on a chair next to the bed and takes my hand. He looks tired. He needs a shave. Billy stands on the other side of the bed. He touches my forehead. All these machines and tubes attached to my arms and everything hurts.

One of the doctors, the young one, moves in and Billy steps away.

"You're going to be okay now," he says.

When was I not going to be okay? Where's Anthony? Is he

here? Why so many nurses doing things to me. I just want to sleep. I want to get back to that other place. Am I talking aloud? God, what pain! Please let me sleep.

Mark says, "I brought the Grieg piano concerto CD that you like. Would you like me to put the headphones on so you can listen to it?" Oh yes. It's a favorite. I was given that record album for my 10th birthday. I used to listen to it again and again, especially when I was hurt or unhappy. I still do. I lie back and let the music take me back to that place.

I was talking to such a nice doctor there. He had an accent. Norwegian, I think. Can't remember his name. Andersen? I open my eyes. It's the German doctor who stands over me.

"Good morning, Sandra. I have good news." He starts to reel off new percentages. I shake my head, close my eyes. I don't want to hear them. "How's the pain? Need more medication?"

No, I just need to get out of here.

"Sandra, I want you to breathe into this, hard enough to raise the ball. Can you do that? Try." A nurse is raising a device to my mouth, a clear plastic tube with a little ball inside. "Mom, see, you take a breath and then blow into this." Billy is showing me how. Mark says something to Billy. "She has to," Billy says. "She's got to strengthen her lungs. Try, Mom."

I am fully back now. They tell me I've been here two days. Today they want me to stand up. How do you stand with only one kidney? Walk around with one kidney? Won't I list to one side?

Margery comes in with a huge box of cookies. "For the nurses," she explains. "They'll be glad to come in." Julie smiles. She's stopped meditating, so I guess I'm out of the woods, so to speak. Out of the woods and into the bathroom with just one kidney. A nurse holds the IV stands and rolls it along with me; another nurse holds my arm. They want me to pee. With one kidney? How does that work? There's some sort of bag attached to me full of blood. My sons shouldn't have to see this.

. . . .

I'm home. Recovery, in spite of the surgeon's promises, is agonizingly slow. Besides the pain, there's the indignity of having a catheter and urine bag tinged with blood attached to me, which has to be emptied every few hours. Mark is staying with me; he does this with amazing good grace. Billy's on food patrol, bringing soups and pasta every day. For some reason, what I crave is fettuccini Alfredo and wilted spinach, which either Mark or Billy picks up at Farfalla, the Italian restaurant down the street. I gather this must be because the person whose blood I got was an Italian gourmand.

One night my dreams take me back to a place I saw while under anesthesia. When I wake I can't seem to grab hold of it to remember. The harder I try the more the images slip away. I give up and open my eyes. It is dawn. In the gray light, I see vases filled with flowers, baskets of fruit, a teddy bear, cards: a *mis en scene* for a sickroom There is a sickroom smell.

I realize it's the wilting flowers and the overripe fruit that are giving off that smell. Who was it who compared cancer to rotting fruit, a condition of stagnation and fermentation in the lymph fluids? I've been lying here too long. I sit up. I've got to get some air in this room and into me. Painfully, I stand. Dragging the catheter bag, I make my way to the window and slide it open. My torso's on fire, knife-like pains shoot through me. I almost cry out, but I stop myself. Mark is sleeping in the next room in my office turned guest room, and I don't want to alarm him and have him come rushing into the room. I breathe the cool fresh air deep into where the pain is.

The pale morning moon is about to disappear behind the hills to make way for the sun. Watching it I begin to remember. In my dream state, powered by anesthesia, I had built a bridge and floated across it, making my own shamanic journey. I left the land of hurt and wounds and sickness and arrived in a place of total healing. In that place I was given something. A piece of that wisdom I had been searching for all these twelve moons. How do I find that piece again?

I think back to that first oncologist who told me my disease was incurable, and without once looking me straight in the eye said that the best I could expect was to live another three to five years. Dr. Darling with the Hollywood teeth cut that to three. All right, I took their medicine, now what? I gave them a kidney, now what? Do I now live with the sword of Damocles over my head for the next three years waiting for it to fall, for the proverbial other shoe to drop?

No, because I saw something, something about my healing, my true healing. It lies not in the laps of the gods, not even the white-coated ones. It lies within me. It's for me to refuse the sword and the other damn shoe. I have rendered unto Caesar that which is Caesar's. I have given my pound of flesh (well, 120 grams to be exact). I turn now to the healers.

Where do I start? First, I want Charley back. Mark agrees

to walk her and feed her. Chris brings her. Charley flies into my arms and covers my face with monkey kisses. Chris and I get to talking about healers. She knows some that are new to me. We decide we will get to work soon and compile a list.

I have remembered.

Transportado

O child of time

Time is in your body

As the turtle that flows

Moon is in your body

As the time that knows

Look inside the moon and

Tell me what you see

The Turtle and the Tree

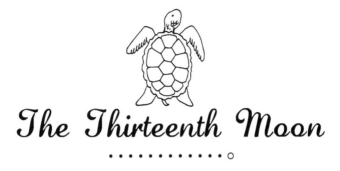

The Thirteenth Moon

· · · · · · · · · · · ○

In no hurry to get back to bed, I slip a CD into the player and linger a while longer at the window. My eyes fall on the turtle collection on the table next to the lamp. I pick up the largest, a beautiful one carved of dark mahogany and bring it to the couch where I sit curled, turning it over in my hand.

"Thirteen scales on old Turtle's back," the man in the Pine Ridge Trading Post said, "one for each month of the year. Lakota moons do not follow today's twelve-month calendar. Lakota moons follow the seasons: spring, summer and fall each have three moons, winter has four. The month of two moons, that you call the blue moon, is to us the thirteenth moon." He points to the turtle's back. "These thirteen scales hold the key to the mysteries of the moon," He looked up at me and added, "or those who know how to look."

I sit, feet propped up on the couch, and listen to the Grieg piano concerto, letting my mind settle into stillness. After a while, I reach that pure place where I can no longer tell the difference between the dream state and wakefulness. It is the space outside time, where poems and books are written and pictures are painted. In music it is the silence between the notes. In writing it is the unsaid word, the white on the page. This is the place where healing happens, the place of the Thirteenth Moon.

The Tibetans have a turtle story too. It is called The Story of the Blind Turtle. Imagine a blind turtle, roaming the depths of an ocean the size of the universe. Up above it floats a wooden ring tossed to and fro on the waves. Every hundred years the turtle comes to the surface just once. To be born a human being is more difficult than for that turtle to surface with its head poking through the wooden ring.

In my ocean in this time-space I know as the Thirteenth Moon, I poke my head through a wooden ring and look around me. The sea that stretches before me is sapphire, the sky cerulean blue. A few clouds glide overhead, regal, swan-like. Land lies not too far in the distance. Holding onto the wooden ring, I kick my feet and head for it. When I feel I can swim the rest of the way, I let go of the wooden ring and watch as it drifts and bobs its way back out to sea to wait for the next blind turtle, perhaps.

Soon, I catch a wave and let it carry me the rest of the way to shore. I stand and wade through the shallow water to pink-white sands dazzling in the midday sun. It's so warm that by the time I cross the beach to the road my light cotton pants and white shirt are already dry. I note that I seem to have been born into this human life fully clothed, except for shoes.

I know this place. This is the place I went to while I was under anesthesia during the operation. I was looking for the white light, I remember, when I came upon this land. I have found my way back to it. I've been, as Bebeto promised, *transportado!* The road of ground coral scratches the bottom of my feet. I wish for sandals. At that very moment, I spot a dark-skinned woman sitting beneath a canopy of dried grass weaving strips of leather into sandals. Next to her is a sign, Baskets $2, Hats $3, Sandals $4. Automatically, I start to reach into my pockets but quickly realize I have no money. The woman smiles. "That's okay," she says, "you can pay me later. With a cool drink like lemonade or maybe an iced tea."

I walk on, but I do not see a single tourist shop, bar, hotel or restaurant, not a single car or taxi or a moped anywhere, not a pharmacy or fast food place or gas station. I come to an intersection and see a signpost with a directory:

Health Food Store
Organic Market
Herbs and Homeopathic Shop
Tea House
Juice bar
(I make a mental note to pick up a drink for the sandal lady. But wait, if I have no money, how will I pay?)
The Carapace is carved into a wooden arrow pointing in the opposite direction (I make another mental note to find out what that is.)
Healers and Hospital 1 km. (Healers and Hospital? I have to check that out.)

I pass a few people on bicycles who smile and wave, a dog

sleeping on a doorstep, a few barefoot children playing jump rope. I stop and turn and look again. Two of the children are bald, one wearing a cap, the other a kerchief. Cancer children.

I walk to the hospital which sits at the top of a hill, a two-story limestone building with tall black-shuttered windows. I enter through oak-paneled double doors into a lobby that looks like a small European hotel with comfortable chairs and sofas, tables decorated with fresh flowers, and everywhere tall ferns and palms in blue and white cachepots. Strains of Chopin fill the air, just as I would have it.

Behind the reception desk sits a pleasant looking woman wearing a crisp white shirt. She smiles, greets me and asks how she might help me. I don't know where to begin. Curious to know how cancer is treated here in the Land of Healers, I ask if the hospital has an oncology department.

"Yes," she says. "It's at the end of that hall, last door on the right. Just walk right in. Someone will be glad to help you."

The waiting room is small; the seven or eight seats are all occupied. What strikes me first is that every one of the patients have all their hair. More than that, their faces are bright, not pale and ashen. And they look happy. At the desk is a nurse who looks up and asks if I have an appointment. I explain that I am just a tourist, curious about the facility. "That's fine," she says, "you're welcome to wait. One of the doctors should be free shortly to answer any questions." A white-haired man stands to give me his seat. I thank him, but politely decline. He insists. As I take the seat, he asks if I am a patient. I tell him I am not.

"I am," he says. "I came here six months ago with prostate

cancer. I had just gotten married to my high school sweetheart I hadn't seen in 50 years. No way I was going to ruin my honeymoon," he smiles sweetly. "If you get my drift."

I smile back. I get the drift.

"So the doc changed my diet, put me on some herbs and supplements and sent me down there to *The Carapace* to see a microbiologist, Dr. Robert Young, who put me on a protocol to alkalize my body. Cancer needs an acid condition to survive, he said. He had me drinking a gallon of alkalized water every day and guzzling green drinks besides. Last week my PSA levels were back to normal. He's going to run tests today—blood, saliva and hair tests—and then I'm done."

"How did you find this place? I mean how did you get here?"

A woman's voice answers, "I think I dreamed myself here." She is sitting across from us knitting. She is young, early thirties, perhaps. Her dark hair is pulled back in a pony tail and she wears horned-rimmed glasses attached to a beaded chain. "I had a tumor in my stomach the size of a grapefruit. My students thought I was pregnant. I had the tumor removed surgically then I came here to complete the healing process.

"I was supposed to start chemo a few weeks after the surgery, but I had no insurance. I'm not a praying sort of person but that brought me to my knees. One day, I wandered into a museum; I don't know why, and came upon an 18th century painting of a landscape by an unknown artist, the most beautiful landscape I had ever seen with sea and sand, thatched-roof houses, white birds flying overhead. It was a place of such peace I couldn't get it out of my mind.

"For days I kept visualizing that painting. I could see myself in it, walking along that beach, coming to that road, walking past the thatched roof houses. At night before I'd go to sleep, I'd see it in my mind's eye, and the memory would calm me. One night I had a dream—I couldn't remember it exactly, only that I was finding my way here." She pauses, smiles. "When I woke up, I was here."

I was about to tell her how it happened to me when the double doors swing open and a man with a familiar looking face steps out. "Here's my doctor!" the woman says.

The doctor waves to her, then stops at the desk. He turns and comes toward me, hand extended. "I am Dr. Andersen. I understand you'd like to speak to me? I'm on a break. If you'd like to join me for a cup of tea in the cafeteria, then perhaps I can show you around. Hi, Jean, see you in a few minutes, okay?"

"Sure. Take your time."

As we walk down the hall, the doctor says, "I see you've met some of my patients."

"I think I've met you before, too. Strange. I think you came to me while I was under anesthesia, you and this place. Is that possible?"

He smiles. "Everything is possible."

The two children I'd seen on the road come running past us, each carrying a tiny kitten. "Look, Doctor Mike. Look what we found! We're taking them to the kid's ward."

"Ask the nurse to give you some warm milk."

"I saw those children on my way over here and wondered why they were bald. Do you give chemo treatments?"

"No, they had already had chemo. They're here to get strong again, same as you."

A man and woman stop him to ask where the Healer's Wing is. "Straight ahead," Dr. Andersen says, "elevator on the left."

We pass what at first looks like an emergency room, but when I stop to look I see that each and every patient is attended by a triage nurse who is sitting as he or she makes an evaluation. I notice that no patient is alone.

"How can the hospital afford such a large staff?" I ask.

"They're all volunteers, not trained nurses. People who come here come because either they've had conventional treatment and want to complete their healing or because they do not choose conventional medicine at all. We don't believe in fighting cancer, we believe in healing it. We use many different modalities.

"Both here at the hospital and at The Carapace, all services are provided free, made possible by donations from our wealthy friends. Since there is no insurance here and we have no ties to pharmaceutical companies, we are free to help everyone who finds their way here."

Music is floating out from one of the rooms just ahead, beautiful choral music. I look questioningly at Dr. Andersen, who points to the partly open door. I peek in. It is a meeting room. People are sitting quietly, eyes closed. A sign on a stand reads: Bruno Groening, Circle of Friends. Medical Scientific Group.

"What's going on?" I ask in a whisper.

"Physicians from around the world are presenting documentation to our staff of the healings that have occurred as a result of the teachings of Bruno Groening."

I remember then. Chris told me about him. He was a famous healer who died many years ago, yet somehow his energy continues to be available to heal anyone who learns to do a certain kind of meditation according to his teachings.

The music has stopped. Dr. Andersen motions to me, and we slip in quietly and stand at the back. A woman is speaking about the spontaneous healings that have occurred as a result of doing *einstellen*.

Dr. Andersen whispers, "*Einstellen* means tuning in to the healing stream. The woman speaking is Dr. Lucia Colizoli, a psychiatrist who has been leading *Einstallen* groups for several years."

"How is that done?"

He nods in the direction of the man who is speaking.

In a heavy German accent he is telling of a spontaneous healing of a stroke victim that occurred recently in Frankfurt. The healing resulted from attending several meetings, listening to the teachings of Bruno Groening, and tuning in daily to the stream of vital energy.

As we leave, Dr. Andersen explains. "These doctors have been documenting cases of fully regained health for people who had been suffering from every imaginable disease—mental illness, stroke, arthritis, blindness, deafness, cancer, addiction, even financial problems."

"Just by meditating?"

"No, not just any kind of meditation. It's more specific. There are Bruno Groening meetings over at The Carapace; you might try to attend one."

I glance sideways at him, skeptically. I remember where I am. "Okay. As you said, everything is possible."

We come to the cafeteria and get in line. Dr. Andersen asks if I'd like tea. Remembering I have no money (is there a way to bring money to this land?), I say "No thanks, just water would be fine."

We take a table at the window. He has brought two cups and a teapot, and shares his tea with me. In the distance I can see a huge expanse of very blue ocean that seems to stretch out forever. Overhead the sky is crystal clear. I have a million questions. "What exactly is The Carapace?" I ask. "A turtle shell, isn't it?"

"Yes. The word 'carapace' is derived from Spanish and Italian and means 'dear peace or the 'face of peace.' It's a converted house with offices, meeting rooms, and rooms for people to stay when they come for workshops or retreats."

"You mean I can come back here? How do I do that?"

"The same way you got here this time." He pauses, peers at me over his glasses, "with the force of your intention." He looks at his watch. "I'm afraid I have to get back. Would you like to visit the Healers Wing? I can walk you down there, it's on my way."

"Healers Wing, of course." I follow him down another long corridor, my new leather sandals squeaking on the tile floor. I notice the walls are lined with framed travel posters: Montana, Connecticut, California, Germany, Italy, Norway, Denmark. Why these particular places, I wonder? When we come to a pair of glass doors, the doctor inserts a card and they slide open.

Inside is a nurse's station. A woman in a crisp white uniform looks up.

"Any particular healer you'd like to see?" Dr. Andersen asks.

I shake my head. "Anyone who's free."

"How about Dr. Jim MacKimmie?"

"But he's in Montana" I say, puzzled. "Isn't he?" Even in a dream isn't he still a thousand miles away?

"Third door on the right," The nurse says, pointing with her pencil.

The doctor grins. "She'll page me when you're finished," he says.

Jim's name is on the door. I knock.

"Come on in, Sandy." The voice is muffled. I can't tell where it's coming from.

"Jim?"

I pass through the door to another hallway, this one smaller and much narrower. At the far end of the hallway, there is another door that is heavier with a metal industrial-type opener. I push it open.

The sunlight is blinding. I have to shade my eyes.

"Over here." There he stands, smiling, at the door of his log cabin, his snowy hair a halo around his head. Beside him his lovely wife, Andrea, beckons me to come in.

"How did I get *here*?" I ask, stunned.

Jim laughs. "You knew the way." He leads me past his makeshift cat dormitory, which occupies part of what was once a garage but now serves as a storeroom. The living room doubles as his treatment room. Andrea excuses herself, explaining that she's working at the computer answering Jim's hundreds of emails. Through the window I spot a family of deer grazing behind the house. A large bird swoops past.

"Here," Jim says, patting the treatment table as he always did. "Let's see how you're doing." Sitting on the stool behind my head, he places his hands just above my face, sending waves of warmth surging through me.

"Jim, I don't understand," I say. "Am I really here?"

"Only if you're in the moment. If you get out of the moment and into your head, you won't be. Just breathe now. Don't think."

Jim's non-negotiable instructions about diet and nutrition come to mind—no coffee, sugar (including chocolate—ouch!) or milk products, and plenty of clean water, exercise and sunshine—are sprinkled with quotes from Shakespeare, Aristotle, Goethe, and his mentor, who he refers to as the "Old Man" and has been dead some fifty years.

"The Old Man said the heart's inner wisdom will guide and direct your life perfectly; it's the mind that's the troublemaker. Your mind is so proud of its great knowledge. Your soul, certain of its destiny, waits patiently for you to discover the true knowledge, the wisdom that abides within your heart. The heart leads; you must follow."

He brings the stool around to the foot of the table and holds my feet.

"I've been having some joint pains which started around Christmas," I tell him, "and my back bothers me now and then."

He has me sit up and works the muscles in my shoulders and back and finishes with a series of small chop-like pats.

"You're doin' fine," he says. "Really great. Just go with the flow, that's all. Real simple if you don't drive yourself crazy thinking.

Stay in the moment and out of your head."

"But what's causing the pains?" I don't tell him what it is I'm afraid of. I don't know why I don't tell him.

"Just toxins working their way out of the body. Nothing sinister. When you're looking for an answer, don't look here," he taps me on the forehead. "The answer's here," he taps my chest, "in your heart."

As I get up and put on my sandals, I'm thinking: How do you find answers in the heart?

"If you watch your thoughts," Jim says, "you'll see how insane they are. They're always either in the future or in the past. The heart though, stays in the sacred-now moments, loving acceptance of everything and everyone right now in this very moment. So as you see, so shall it be.

"And remember, drink lots of water."

He walks me to the door and we hug. "You're doin' just great," he says. "Energy's really flowing now. See you soon!"

I open the door, but I'm not outside under Montana's big blue sky; I'm back in the hospital corridor. I lean my back against the closed door and think: Okay, behind this door is Montana. What's behind all those other doors? I cross the hall, intending to open one, when Dr. Andersen appears.

"Looking for me?" he asks.

"Actually, I was looking for Germany."

"Germany the country?" He gives me a baffled sort of laugh and hands me a bottle of water.

I thank him. "Yes, I'd like to see Paulo. I was wondering if he was behind one of those other doors."

"I don't know. Let's find out."

I follow him to the desk. The doctor peers over at the book. "I don't see his name. He might be over at The Carapace. Do you know Melissa Deedon?" he asks me.

"Yes, I do. Melissa's here? I haven't seen her since she moved back East. To Connecticut, I thought."

The nurse says, "I see she's at an event, but she ought to be free soon."

"How do I find her?" I ask. "Which door?"

"She's on the second floor," the nurse replies, "that elevator on the left."

I step into an old fashioned elevator that reminds me of the ones in downtown New York with heavy iron gates that clang shut and start with a sudden lurch. I realize I've forgotten to ask where I go when I get to the second floor when the elevator groans to a stop and the gates open--onto a country lane!

Cool, fresh air mingled with the smell of pine greets me as I head down a winding lane lined on each side with stone walls. The houses are white clapboard with black or green shutters and shaded by oak trees, red maples, and elm. I am in Connecticut. No crowded airport, no long security lines, I am here, just like that, in Connecticut. I love this Land of Healers.

In the distance I spot what looks at first like a small black dot streaking toward me. Then I see it's a puppy, ears flying, tail straight. It's *my puppy!* Charley leaps up onto on her hind legs and frantically paws me. I bend down to pick her up, ignoring the pain that shoots across my back. How did she get here? She gives my face several licks then squirms to be put down.

Off she goes back down the lane, making a sharp right turn into a driveway. "Charley!" I call after her, but she's off on some mission of her own.

A sign reads, Fairfield Unity Church. I follow Charley around to a field behind the church where a crowd is gathered. Dogs are everywhere and cats too, and birds, goats, pigs. I ask a little girl holding a rabbit in her arms what's going on.

"We're having an animal blessing," she says. "Melissa is doing a healing of all the animals."

Of course! I remember hearing that she did animal healings, as well as healings on people. I had met Melissa in California a few years ago. She's blonde, blue-eyed in her 40s, an unlikely looking shaman. Word of her astounding healings is heard throughout the country and in Europe.

I spot her standing in a semicircle surrounded by a crowd of noisy children and barking dogs. When she opens her arms in greeting and begins a prayer, a hush falls over the field. Children grow silent; dogs, including Charley, lie down next to their owners. From my vantage point I cannot quite make out all the words but I gather Melissa is bestowing a blessing on all the animals, and I hear her command that all creatures be healed. This goes on for ten or fifteen minutes.

Afterward, Charley runs right up to Melissa and stands on her hind legs to get her attention. I make my way through the crowd and watch as she kneels and cups Charley's head in her hands. "Who've we got here?" she asks. I introduce myself and Charley, and remind her that we met in California.

"I do remember you," Melissa says. "We met through Judith

Prager. You're visiting someone here in Fairfield?"

I explain I'm visiting healers in various places. I stop short of telling her I got here by magic elevator.

"Can you hang around a while?" she asks. "We can go over there and sit," she points to a couple of chairs under the shade of a giant oak, "and catch up."

Charley runs off with a Jack Russell, and they take turns chasing each other. Melissa explains she likes to take a day off now and then from doing her people healings to work with animals. "Pleasant switch from two-leggeds to four-leggeds."

A young man brings us a tray of lemonade. A cool breeze rustles the leaves, I breathe deeply, filling my lungs with clean fresh New England air, a world away from Los Angeles smog.

"You're looking great," she says.

I start to tell her about my recent bout with cancer, but she stops me. "That's in the past. It's important to let it go now. I know, because right after I got married and moved to Germany with my husband--almost ten years ago, I was diagnosed with cancer. I was given two months to live."

"My god, what did you do?"

"I remembered watching my Grandma die of pancreatic cancer when I was a girl. I swore then I would never die like that. When the doctor laid out a protocol for me, I decided not to follow it. I chose not to do anything. I just let go of all fear of dying. If I was going to die, so be it. I would live in the moment.

"Then one night my Grandma came to me in a vivid dream. She told me not to worry, that I would be healed. The next day I made a decision. I packed up and went home to Pennsylvania. I slept. For more than a month I slept. After that, one day I woke up and the pain was gone, and I knew it was true. I was healed. I knew I had work to do."

"Melissa, how did you know? I mean that was quite a leap of faith."

"No, no, not faith. I just *knew*. I knew with every fiber of my being that I was well. That once I let go of the fear of illness and dying, my own body's ability to heal would take over. It was not a miraculous healing or anything like that, I just let go. When I did, in that instant, that *second*, I was healed."

Just then a little boy of four or five dressed in overalls comes toward us, tugging at a goat. "He's not a good goat," the boy declares. "He won't do anything I tell him."

Melissa nods sympathetically and, kneeling, whispers something to the goat. Then to the little boy, she says, "Maybe you need to let him be a goat, not try to make him a doggie." She looks at the goat. "Try giving him apples."

Smiling, she turns to me. "You have work to do, too." She gives me a quick hug and heads off with the little boy.

I start down the lane, Charley bounding along beside me, when it occurs to me: *I have no idea where I'm going.* How am I supposed to get back? I assume I'm still in Connecticut. What do I do now?

I sit on a tree stump. I guess what Melissa was showing me is what I've been hearing from scientists and biologists like Bruce Lipton. Bruce said "The body knows what it needs to heal itself… The mind shapes the body, opposite of what conventional allopathic medicine believes—that the body shapes itself. But first we have to take a big giant step back and realize that we create this reality. That's the bottom line of physics. Physics states that the observer creates the reality."

I teased him about that. "You mean, just like the bumper stickers say?"

He laughed too, and said, "Yes, exactly."

Melissa healed herself of cancer by letting go of all fear, which allowed her body to heal itself. Is that really possible?

Suddenly, I realize Charley's disappeared. I whistle and call her. No Charley. Across the road is a thicket, where a large bush is rustling. She might have gone in there after something, a rabbit maybe. Making my way through the tangle of prickly branches I spot her. She's sniffing and scratching, whining at something—a door. Next to the door is a doorbell. I peer closer. It's not a doorbell but a button. I press it. The door slides open to an elevator—clever, clever Charley. I press number 1 and the gate clangs shut. I scoop Charley up in my arms and kiss her monkey nose. "Good girl," I say. The gate squeaks open and I am once again in the hospital corridor.

"Oh, hi," a woman in scrubs calls out, "visiting pets go to the Children's Ward down that hall and turn left. Can't miss it."

Obediently, I follow the directions. When I see balloons tied to a doorknob, I open the door. Children are in wheelchairs or in beds with their legs or arms in casts, or sitting up in bed playing video games, some holding cats or dogs on their laps. I observe that none of the children look terribly sick, just in need of repair.

A nurse takes Charley from me and asks if I can come back for her in a couple of hours. Charley has already made a friend.

A little girl in a wheelchair is holding her and stroking her head. Charley's tail is going a mile a minute. I leave her and go in search of Dr. Andersen. I find him at the entrance to a gift shop where he is buying flowers. "These are for a woman," he says, "an oncology patient."

Tagging along, I follow the doctor to a door. He knocks on the door then opens it. Lying in bed, head just slightly elevated by two pillows, her face ghostly white, is a woman who looks vaguely familiar. She manages a smile when she sees the flowers, then looks at me. "Hi," she says.

It takes a minute, then I remember. She's the woman from the cancer clinic at Norris, the one with the funny ring tone on her cellphone. I also remember she kept having all those treatments for the same exact cancer I had. She's the same one who said the words that stuck in my head like some jingle for Alka Seltzer, *It always comes back.*

Perplexed, I turn to Dr. Andersen.

"Felicia has come here to make peace," he says, "and get ready."

"But this is the Land of Healers!" I exclaim. "Surely...."

Felicia shakes her head. "This is my healing," she says. "Hard as I tried, deep down I knew I couldn't beat it. I knew it from the day I was diagnosed."

I don't understand. Incredulous, I ask Dr. Andersen, "What about all these healers? Can't one of them help her?"

Felicia answers, "They tried, but it was too late for me. By the time I got here my cancer was too far gone." Her head sinks into the pillow. "Dr. Andersen can explain." She closes her eyes and smiles weakly. "Tell her the lightbulb joke."

Dr. Andersen takes my arm. We leave quietly. I turn to him, tears half of anger and outrage welling up. "I don't get it," I say. "Why can't she be healed?"

"Do you know how many healers it takes to change a lightbulb?" he asks.

I shake my head. "No, dammit it, I don't know."

"One, but the lightbulb has to really *want* to change."

I don't laugh. I don't even smile.

"Sandy, you can't heal without changing," he says. "Felicia found that out too late, I'm afraid."

Dr. Andersen watches me carefully as my countenance grows dark and grim.

We stand silently for a moment. Then he says, "You still haven't figured it out yet, have you?"

"Figured what out?"

"What it was that caused your cancer."

I shake my head and shrug. "I don't know," I answer dismally. "Too many French fries?"

"I mean the root causes, the emotional factors: The shocks and traumas that were never released from the body, old resentments and self-judgments, and fear. Fear gives off toxins, you know, chemicals that weaken the immune system."

"I'm not sure I care how I got cancer. People get cancer same as people get MS or Parkinson's or ALS. It happens. Earthquakes happen, tornados happen, tsunamis happen." My voice rises, I'm trying hard to fight back tears. Felicia's relapse is making me doubt everything—this place, these healers. My back starts to hurt.

"Why don't you go down to The Carapace? I think you may find some old friends there."

"No, I think I'll go home," I reply. I need to sort all this out. "Maybe some other time."

Dr. Andersen looks directly into my eyes. The kind of hard, meaningful look Bebeto gives me. "Sandy, listen to me," he says. "There is no other time."

· · · · · · · · · · · ·

The three-story clapboard house sits at the opposite end of the road from the hospital at the bottom of the hill and occupies an acre of land, most of it behind the building. A long sweeping veranda faces the front with wicker furniture, chairs, chaise lounges, tables arranged in seating groups like a country club setting. Around back is a round structure covered with canvas, which I instantly recognize as a Native American sweat lodge. Nearby is a tent surrounded by benches, probably used as a changing room. Just beyond that is a children's playground shaded by a huge oak.

I walk around front and climb the steps to the veranda. A directory is next to the door:

Trauma therapist — Judith Simon Prager
Cellular biologist — Dr. Bruce Lipton
Chiropractor — Dr. Stephen Ward
Acupuncturist — Ken Kobayashi
CranialSacro therapist — Sandra Cappeli
Nutritionist — Dr. Mary Hardy
Qi Qong Energy — Michael Mohoric

Microbiologist — Dr. Robert Young
Group Healing — Bruno Groening Circle of Friends

I know these people, some I have even worked with. I open the front door and enter a hallway with a line of doors bearing nameplates. Judith's is the first. Remembering she's in China doing crisis training for counselors dealing with the victims of the earthquake, I slip a note under her door telling her to call me when she gets back.

The next office is Dr. Stephen Ward's, a chiropractor whose unusual practice is called Spinal Column Stressology, a mind-boggling skill involving reading spines. Like a phrenologist reads heads and an iridologist reads eyes, Dr. Steve can not only see a patient's health—emotional and physical—he can see the patient's entire history from birth in the curve of the spine. More than that, once he finds the problem, he fixes it!

I had been to his office in Long Beach a few times about my back (which he fixed in three quick adjustments), and to my astonishment, he began to reel off my health problems, including the big one which he spotted right off.

He's a big guy, over six feet tall, and strong and bald as Mr. Clean. He put a couple of X-rays up on a lightbox and showed me the difference between a normal, efficient spine and one with a left curve, which is what I and most cancer profiles have. He explained that all illnesses have a particular spinal pattern in common. I must call and make an appointment to see him again.

At the end of the hall is Bruce Lipton's office. I had spoken to him some months earlier when I was deep into my research, and we agreed to meet sometime when he was not traveling and lecturing.

His door is ajar. I stick my head in. When I see he's on the phone I start to back out, but he motions for me to wait.

"Sorry," I say when he hangs up. "I didn't mean to disturb."

"Not at all." Bruce stands and invites me to sit down. Bearded, wearing a Hawaiian shirt, he smiles broadly. We begin to chat, and I wind up telling him about Felicia. I tell him how her words "It always comes back" have haunted me, and now here she is dying in of all places the Land of Healers!

"But look at what she said," he replies. "That's her belief, don't you see? Don't allow her truth to become your truth. You must not download her program and decide therefore one day you must also have a recurrence."

"Are you saying I can prevent a recurrence with my belief?"

"When cancer recurs it's because there were issues that precipitated the first one that were never resolved. There are people who have a remission, it goes away, and it never comes back. Somewhere in the process, they have profoundly learned about whatever it was that caused the problem. Yet, other people may think, oh this is what the problem was, and they try to work it out rationally. They later find the cancer has come back. That's because that rational approach didn't get to what the problem was."

"So by then it's too late?" I ask, thinking of Felicia. "Is it already a runaway train?"

Bruce nods. "Sometimes when the acceleration has gone too fast, at that point it's hard to get your hands around it and hold it back."

I think I'm beginning to see something. Felicia is my dreaded doppelganger. From the first moment I met her in the waiting room at Norris and we laughed about our identical wigs, I felt a connection. Another link was the ring tone on her cellphone that made us laugh, because when she told me it was a song by a former Eagle, I thought she was talking about a football player. Then, some months later, when I saw her so sick after many rounds of chemo, I found out we both had the same diagnosis. My doppelganger believed absolutely that her cancer would come back. It did, and now she is dying, just as she knew she would. Could that possibly be true? "Are our beliefs that powerful?" I ask Bruce again.

"Yes. Your own thoughts and your own energy and your own beliefs are energy fields. They can turn things on and off all your life. In your conscious mind are the desires, wishes, all you want from life. In your subconscious mind are the programs." He pauses, looks at me. "Got it?"

I nod. "So far."

"Problem is, the conventional person thinks he's running his life with his conscious desires. Science has demonstrated, neuroscience, that the conscious mind only operates about five percent of the day. That means that 95% of the day, all operations of the machine—body, behavior, action—are controlled by the subconscious mind. The subconscious mind has programs that it got from other people, programs that do not necessarily support what the conscious mind desires.

"Once you identify what you do want, you have to then identify the beliefs that are preventing you from getting those things.

We need to recognize the power of our own thoughts. But the real issue is, our programming has inevitably undermined us in every way possible, disempowering us from believing that. When you become disempowered, then you become a victim. When you become a victim, you necessitate a rescuer, and you bring into play a whole industry to come and help the victim that never really was a victim."

"I see," I said, but then as I wandered on down the hall, the question that was still hanging in my mind: How exactly does one go about changing one's beliefs? After one has identified those beliefs that undermine, what then? A set of instructions is needed here.

I pass the Yoga Studio, the Massage Room, Chiropractor, Healers Suite; but, nowhere do I see a place for changing beliefs--an office perhaps or a studio equipped with a large container for dingy old beliefs and beside it another for bright shiny new ones.

I once had a belief change. I think of it as my potato chip moment. It was in July, when everyone I knew seemed to be away somewhere. I woke one morning with a dull, burning pain in my abdomen, the very place and the very pain I felt that first sent me to the doctor. I was on the verge of panic, but not wanting to place a call to one of the doctors, I decided to call Bebeto instead.

"I'm scared, Bebeto. I think it's come back." I tried to sound calm.

"No, it hasn't," he said.

"But," I proceeded to describe the symptoms.

"By any chance are you constipated?"

"Well, come to think of it, yes I am a little."

"Take a tablespoonful of castor oil. See if that helps."

"Yuck, Bebeto, I'm not that constipated."

"You prefer to think you're dying?"

I went to the drugstore and bought the stuff. At the checkout I spotted potato chips, not the fancy health food kind, but my favorite, plain old Lay's Ruffles. Understand, potato chips to cancer patients trying to rebuild their health are on the Forever Forbidden list, along with chocolate, coffee, candy of any kind, white bread and In-N-Out Burgers. If I was going to have to swallow castor oil, for god's sake, I needed something for the aftertaste. "I do not believe these potato chips will hasten my demise," I announced to anyone who happened to be listening.

Once in the car, doors locked, I opened the Lays, just to inhale the salty greasiness of them and I lost control. I finished half the bag before I got home. I did not feel guilty, I felt liberated. For the first time in seven months, I felt like a perfectly normal person having some potato chips on a summer afternoon. By the time I got into the building, up the elevator and into my apartment, the pain was gone, all trace of it, and without the castor oil. I remember calling Judith and laughing.

"See?" she said, "What you experienced was a spontaneous healing triggered by a shift in focus and followed by an act of empowerment in which you took full responsibility for yourself and did exactly as you pleased. The shift in focus was a quantum leap from fear to your own personal bliss, which in your case happened to be a bag of potato chips.

"What it proves is that consciousness precedes matter, and matter follows mind. It *all* originates with thought. Every thought has a physiological reaction and creates chemicals that harm or heal. The thoughts that will keep you well are thoughts of love and gratitude."

Love and gratitude. That reminds me of something I'm forgetting. I become aware of music coming from one of the rooms, that same beautiful choral music I heard back in the hospital. A man and a woman come up behind me and open the door. "Coming in?" the woman asks.

"What is it?" I ask.

"It's the community hour for Bruno Groening's Circle of Friends. It's just starting. Please come in."

Ten or twelve chairs are set up in rows. On a table, are photographs of Bruno Groening along with books and pamphlets about his life. I pick one up. The blurb reads:

"...In 1949 one name dominated the headlines: Bruno Groening. Extra editions were printed. There were radio and newsreels reports. A movie was made. Everywhere he appeared tens of thousands flocked to see him from all over Europe and America. Groening became a world event." There is also a letter from Dr. Christiane Northrup, author of several books on healing, praising Groening's Circle, there's another comment from Dr. Carl Simonton, and letters from doctors who have documented healings that occurred as a result of the *heilstrom*, the healing stream.

I take a seat. A man facing the group begins to speak. He talks about the life of Bruno Groening and of the healings that continue to occur whenever groups gather anywhere in the world to listen to his teachings and to absorb the healing stream. He also talks about how today many late-stage cancer patients experience *medically documented* spontaneous healings. He quotes Groening: "You owe it yourself to convince yourself you can heal."

A short film is shown. Footage of Bruno Groening shows a strong, sturdily built man with an intense gaze. The narrator tells us Groening was born in 1906 and died in 1959. "Even as a small boy he was able to absorb and redirect energy from the cosmos. If anyone anywhere focused on this energy and absorbed it with conviction and intention, that person would automatically do *einstallen.* The healing energy would stream through his body. Bruno tells us, 'Nothing is incurable. Nothing.'"

The lights are dimmed. We are told to sit spine-straight, arms and legs uncrossed so that the energy can flow freely through and around us. "Close your eyes, clear your mind and tune in to the healing energy."

At first I feel nothing. After a while I begin to feel warm. A silky warmth begins to flow through me, washing over each cell, each organ, tissue, muscle, every bone in my body. I feel heat in the area of my abdomen. I sit with it, willing myself to experience whatever this is. This intense energy is as great as any I have felt beneath a healer's hands. I feel it move up into my heart, which seems to expand and soften. An indescribable sense of well-being comes over me. I am overwhelmed with a sudden sense of certainty. I might get hit by a truck or fall out of the sky in an airplane or die in any number of ways, but of this I am certain: I am done with this cancer.

The meditation ends with a quote from Bruno Groening: "… there is no illness that cannot be healed, no matter what stage;

there is no pain, no sorrow, no worries. Here there is health, joy, delight and confidence."

Standing outside, I want to laugh out loud. I want to shout *I felt something! I felt the healing energy!* I sat in an uncomfortable wooden chair for two hours and my back doesn't hurt! I bend and stretch without as much as a twinge of pain. I want to tell everyone about this.

Felicia, I have to tell Felicia. I rush back to the hospital, my mind racing. We have to get her down here. She can still change her belief about getting well; I can show her it's not too late, that she too can have this feeling. She can still heal!

On the way I pass a fruit juice stand and suddenly remember the sandal lady! Love and gratitude, of course. I promised her a lemonade as payment for the sandals. On the counter next to the juices are coconuts with a hole in the top for a straw. "I'd like one of those, too," I say. Then I realize I still have no money. "Oh, wait. No, that's all right. Sorry," I say, embarrassed.

The woman points to my chest and smiles. "*Ela é bela!*" She speaks Portuguese. "Is Yemanja, no?"

I frown, put my hand to my chest. I am surprised that I am wearing the charm I had bought in Brazil, a tiny figure of the goddess Yemanja and the title of my novel. I often wore it as a talisman while writing. I had no idea I had it on.

The woman must be Brazilian. "Yes. Yemanja. Do you like it? *Você gosta?*"

Her face lit up, pleased, I suppose, at my effort in Portuguese, and gave me a huge smile.

I took the charm off and handed it to her.

"Oh no. No, Senhora!"

"Yes, please. It's for you. Please take it."

Grinning, the woman took it, kissed it, and fastened it around her neck. "Ooh. *Obrigada,* Senhora. *Obrigada.*" She handed me the lemonade and the coconut and looked around for something else to give me. I laughed and said I couldn't carry any more. She leaned over the counter and kissed me on both cheeks. I hurry to the sandal lady, murmuring my new mantra, "Love and gratitude, love and gratitude..."

I remember something else. In my research I had come across a study done at the Menninger Clinic of 400 patients who had experienced spontaneous remissions from cancer. They discovered that the one unifying thread was that every single person had changed their attitude before their remission occurred. They had moved into a space of being more hopeful, courageous, and positive.

The sandal lady is thrilled. I get another kiss.

Is this the holy grail that researchers at pharmaceutical labs have been spending hundreds of millions dollars every year looking for? It's right here, I want to shout, and all it costs is a lemonade!

Breathless, I run up the stairs to the hospital and dash down the hall to Felicia's room. Dr. Andersen stands outside. I start to call to him to shout my news. Then I see his face. I stop. Tears spring to my eyes.

"She's gone, isn't she?"

He nods.

"Felicia is gone, but she left you something."

I shake my head slowly from side to side.

The doctor holds out a folded piece of paper. "Look at it."

I don't want to see it.

"You must look at it. It is a gift from her to you."

Finally, I take the paper and unfold it. Something rolls to the floor. I bend to pick it up. It's a piece of bright green sea glass.

"Read what she wrote," the doctor insists. "She had a sudden brief spurt of energy and sat up and asked for paper and pencil."

The writing is shaky. It starts at the top of the page and continues around in circles, repeating the words, "*The Matter is the Heart/The Heart is What Matters*" again and again, spiraling into a tiny drawing of a heart.

I read it again, this time aloud, and look at the doctor. "What?"

"Felicia said something about a cellphone ring. Do you know what that means?"

I get it then. Tears start again. "It's the dumb song she had on her phone. 'The Heart of the Matter.' Oh God. But that's what I wanted to tell her—the heart is what matters."

Dr. Andersen puts his arm around my shoulder. "She said the sea glass is a reminder of this place."

He lets me lean my head against him and cry and hands me a tissue. "Go home now, and live your life. Know that you are healed. Know it in a new way, in the deepest part of yourself. It's yours now."

. . . .

I can't seem to find the Children's Ward. I walk up and down the hall looking for the balloons tied to a door, whistling softly. I wonder where all the nurses are. Where is the usual bustle of visitors? "Charley," I call out quietly so as not to disturb the patients. "Charley, come on girl." She lands on my chest with a thud and begins to lick my face. I open my eyes and see Charley's monkey face inches from mine, her huge eyes peering at me.

It takes me a minute. I'm back. I am on the couch, the bright morning sunlight streams through the windows; my cup of tea sits on the coffee table next to yesterday's newspaper; next to it is the wood-carved turtle.

I hear the door to the guest room open, and Mark appears. "Good morning," he says. "How're you feeling today? Want some tea?" He kisses me on the top of my head. "I see you've already had some, let me get you a fresh cup, then I'll take Charley out for a walk." He hands me a stack of mail. "Look through these whenever you feel like it." As I set them down on the table, I notice the card on top is from Norris Cancer Center reminding me that I have a PET/CT scan scheduled for the following week. I look at it for a long time. If the scan were to pick up something, what would I do?

My notebook lies open beside me on the couch. *Go live your life now,* the good doctor said. *Know that you are healed. Know it in a new way.*

I pick up the notebook and reach for a pen. This is my life, my parallel fiction life. Peter had vanished. Had he, like me, vanished into a land on the other side of the looking glass? What was it that the shaman told Sara? *You can't go through the looking glass without getting cut.* The opposite happened to me. I had gone through the looking glass and gotten healed. But not Peter, not yet anyway. His flirtation with the dark mystical powers of the god Exu had left him in shreds. He had no way of knowing that Exu is the god of evil as well as good. Sara will go to the shaman to ask for help, but in her heart she knows it's up to Peter to find his way home, to make his choice, to see that the soul of his art (that he had always sought to find, that he had even made a deal to find) resided inside him, had always been there.

Sara will find Peter, and Peter will choose.

Just as the soul of my healing had always been inside me.

I pick up the card from Norris. *What if?* Would I now have the courage to get up and walk out, find my way back to the Land of Healers, to The Carapace where I might change my belief about the diagnosis? Perhaps do *einstellen* in Bruno Groening's Circle of Friends, absorb the healing energy until whatever it was the scan picked up is gone?

Of one thing I am certain: Healing, true healing, is beyond anything medicine can offer, beyond diet and vitamins and yoga and massage and meditation and pH levels. True healing is something else, something the name of which I do not know. I only know it is there in the Land of Healers and in the hands of certain White Coats, who can heal with White-Coat medicine. Even well-respected medical institutions like Harvard, UCLA, Yale, Stanford, Johns Hopkins, MD Anderson in Houston have begun to incorporate complementary and integrative medicine into their treatment protocols. At the Beth Israel Medical Center in Manhattan, the Dalai Lama met with doctors to discuss how best to merge Western knowledge of brain biology with Eastern wisdom about the nature of the mind.

Looking at the card in my hand summoning me back to the

Land of Cancer, I wonder. Is my resolve any stronger now? Do I have the discipline, the *courage* to quiet the "what ifs" when they jump up and stare me in the face?

I suppose I would go hear what the White Coats have to offer, but then I would try to make my way back to the Land of Healers, ride on alpha waves into my time-space until I land on its shores again.

My yearlong quest—these thirteen moons of seeking—has led me to the deepest part of myself. I learned to look deep inside to pull the fear out by the roots. When I did, I saw how deep those roots really were, how ancient. So that by the time cancer had me in its grip, it already had taken on a life of its own. Had I been alert to the first signals my body and my dreams were sending me that something was way out of balance I might have gotten myself—with the force of my intention—to the Land of Healers. To go there though, to swim those deep waters, fully and with conviction requires courage and a sometimes terrifying belief that must remain unshakable.

I reach down to put on my slippers, imagining for a moment how surprised I would be if I found a pair of brand new hand-made leather sandals instead. And if a piece of bright green sea glass tumbled onto the floor. A thought occurs to me: those sandals and the sandal lady and the sea glass exist inside me now, just like the Land of Healers does. In fact it always has. The way Peter's art had always existed inside him. We just needed to find the way. I look out the window at the sky and see a large majestic cloud soaring overhead. My Old Geezer's sitting up there on that cloud bank, and he's still stopping the rain for me.

I have not been able to change the trajectory of the story of my past, but I think I know now how to rewrite the story of my future.

End

Epilogue
. . . .

I have come to the end of this particular journey, heard its call and heeded it. There will be other calls, I know, to be answered. I will heed them, too, without fear, for I will know now to look into my heart for the answers.

I readily concede that without the intervention of chemotherapy and surgery I might never have made it to the coral-paved road that led me to the Land of Healers. At that time my disease level definitely called for draconian measures. *"Do this and you might live,"* the doctors told me at the time of my diagnosis. I heard that through a prism of fear, and I accepted those words as gospel. After all, when it comes to our health, White Coats rule—or so I thought. I know now too that there are ways to complement White Coat medicine during and especially after treatment. And that had I paid attention to the signs leading up to that diagnosis, known what to do about it, known of the existence of a land where I could get my health back on track before it became a runaway train, I might have avoided such extreme treatment altogether.

Alternative medicine is no longer only found on the other side of the rainbow. It is right here right now. Scientists, researchers and practitioners are working with an array of healing modalities in full view and available for the asking. In response to a growing demand, one in four U.S. hospitals now offer alternative therapies. In fact, according to the American Hospital Association, all 18 hospitals on the *U.S. News and World Report's* "Best Hospitals" list now offers some form of complementary alternative medicine (CAM).

Now after almost five years later, instead of running off to the White Coats whenever I feel a new or familiar pain or (gasp) a lump or bump, which causes my demons to rise up and shout "What if?", I stop a moment and tune into what's going on in my body. "Each patient carries his own doctor inside him," Dr. Albert Schweitzer says. "We are at our best when we give the doctor who resides within each patient a chance to work." The doctors who reside within me are the ones on staff in my private Land of Healers, where I notice the population keeps growing as more and more White Coats open their minds and hearts to have a look at the healing that is happening outside of their conventional paradigm.

· · · · · · · · · · · ·

To those of you dealing with a frightening diagnosis of your own or of a loved one, know that no one, *no one* can know how or what will trigger your healing. Someone said to me, "No wonder you found a way to heal, you met the Dalai Lama." "Right," I said, "I also met a top oncologist who basically told me, forget it, pack it in."

Both voices exist within each of us. One is the voice of love and compassion and belief in our capacity to heal that activates the chemicals of calm and joy. The other is the voice that releases chemicals of fear, adrenaline and cortisols (stress hormones that signal fight or flight) that block the body's natural response to heal itself. You will probably encounter both these voices regardless of what path of treatment you choose.

It was that first voice, the one that speaks of belief in our capacity to heal, that I heeded when my body let me know that modern technology had done its job of reducing the tumor burden. It was now time to let my body's own natural wisdom take over: to clean house, to detox in every way, and to feed the mind with thoughts of beauty, of music and books, a glass of wine with friends at sunset. Time to feed the heart with feelings of love, to find a sense of purpose in life, to make a connection with something larger than oneself (or smaller, like a puppy), and to feed the body equally with high doses of nutrients and peace and happiness.

The most important thing I learned was that to truly heal, one must undergo a transformation at the deepest energy level, at the very core of our emotional and spiritual being. As Bebeto always says, nothing short of complete and total *transportado*. How does one do that? With the mind, as Agre told me in the first days of my diagnosis. Dr. Agre, the most allopathic of allopathic doctors, knew this straight away. Maybe one day, as more and more doctors come to know how great a part the mind plays in healing, they might begin to integrate more alternative complementary medicine into their practices.

· · · · · · · · · · · ·

It was in the time of the Thirteenth Moon, in my time-space I call the Land of Healers that I found my courage. I often think of Felicia and her last message, written to me just before she died: "The matter is the heart; the heart is what matters." I hope she knows there in the land of the spirit how important these words were for me, a gift I will always cherish.

To regain and maintain my health, I have assembled my own team of healers and practitioners: An MD who practices holistic/alternative medicine and who keeps an eye on my lab tests; a naturopath whom I see regularly; a chiropractor who keeps my spine and back muscles strong; a ki healer for energy healing; a craniosacral therapist, and a psychotherapist to help me sort out problems before they take up residence in my body. Once a month, I attend a healing meditation group of Bruno Groening Circle of Friends—two hours of sitting quietly and absorbing the energy stream (heilstrom) with music composed especially for these meetings playing softly in the background.

Now after almost five years later (a year-and-a-half beyond my "expiration date"), I am symptom-free and my lab tests remain normal, officially stamped, "NED" (No Evidence of Disease) and "Durable Remission." In other words (drumroll, please) *gone!*

HANS GRUENN, MD
• • • • • • • • • • • •
EAST MEETS WEST

Dr. Gruenn's offices in West Los Angeles are on the second floor of a small, ivy-covered building. To enter the suite of offices, I walk through a lovely, serene terrace filled with trees and plants and stone urns, and benches for waiting (or to use cellphones). Dr. Gruenn moved to California from his birthplace in Germany twenty years before and has been at the forefront of integrative and preventative medicine ever since. The framed certificates on his wall are from the University of Heidelberg where he completed his residency in internal medicine and his fellowship in psychosomatic medicine. Another is from L.A. County/U.S.C. Hospital where he did his postgraduate training.

Hans Gruenn has no problem straddling both worlds—conventional Western and alternative medicine. In fact he sees no conflict between the two. Each has its place.

"Most chronic diseases," he says, "are caused by the interplay of genetic, biochemical, nutritional, environmental and psycho-social factors. It is not only our genes that make us sick, but also environmental toxins, our diet and lifestyle. If we catch the flu or get a bacterial infection, it is often due to a weak immune system and not just the latest bug. Instead of exclusively treating symptoms, we have to take the relevant underlying factors into account.

"Disease doesn't appear out of nowhere, but is a consequence of a multitude of possible influences. It is well known that various medical and psychosocial risk factors can profoundly impact our health. But just recently we discovered that completely unrecognized by us, our family system and the fate of our ancestors are able to entangle us and make us sick, even generations later. Looking at your health from a trans-generational, 'systemic' perspective provides a powerful and effective tool for self-improvement and healing. If you are able to resolve your family entanglements, you will change the context of your physical and psychological symptoms. Consequently, your symptoms will change or even become superfluous and disappear. If the system changes, so will you—and frequently in ways where change happens naturally and by itself."

MARIE-ANNE BOULARAND, NATUROPATH

· · · · · · · · · · · ·

EVERYTHING THAT DOES NOT RISE INTO CONCIOUSNESS COMES BACK AS DESTINY
CARL JUNG

There is a before. There is an after. All Illnesses, according to the German New Medicine® begin with a shock, a trauma, a precise event in time and space that begins as a sense then becomes a sensation. It enters through our five senses then it attempts to leave the mind/body. If unspoken, it moves into the unconscious, into the biology, into the energy field. This is the foundation of the work of Dr. Rilke Geerd Hamer and the highly controversial and revolutionary German New Medicine®.

Founder and president of the Biodecoding® Institute in Alta Dena, California, French-born Marie-Anne Boularand heads a group of practitioners whose work is based mainly on the discoveries of Dr. Hamer. She is a lovely, soft-spoken young woman (how young she won't say—somewhere in her 30s—not for reasons of vanity; she doesn't celebrate birthdays, doesn't count the years, doesn't buy into the concept of aging.

As a child, Marie-Anne suffered from acute infectious diseases that doctors were unable to cure despite repeated surgeries and treatments, and she developed a rare infection that affected her muscles rendering her unable to move. Worried about the side-effects of the strong medications she was on, medications that were threatening her heart and kidneys, Marie-Anne's mother began to look into alternative medicine— homeopathy and acupuncture and herbs—and took her to see the practitioners. Marie-Anne's health improved rapidly, and within months she was illness free.

As a student, Marie-Ann majored in science, deciding to make natural medicine her life's work. After graduating in Naturopathy, she learned of Dr Hamer's work and knew then the path her work would take.

In 1978, German doctor Ryke Geerd Hamer, a scientific researcher, and head internist of an oncology clinic in Munich who also maintained a thriving practice in Rome, received a call in the middle of the night informing him that his 17-year old son had been shot while on holiday in the Mediterranean. Three months later, his son died. Shortly after, devastated by the catastrophe, Dr. Hamer, who had been in excellent health all of his life, discovered he had testicular cancer. Suspicious of this seeming coincidence, he began to research the personal histories of his many cancer patients. As chief of internal medicine in a gynecology-oncology clinic at Munich University, he had the opportunity to study female patients with cancer and to compare his findings to see if their mechanism was the same as his; if they, too, had suffered some shock, distress or trauma before the onset of illness.

He concluded that a physical event can create a biological conflict-shock that will manifest in a visible transformation in the brain and lead to a measurable change in physical-nervous parameters. These transformations can in turn lead to the development of cancerous growths, ulcerations, necroses and functional disturbances in specific organs of the body. However, if the conflict is resolved, the cancerous or necrotic process can be reversed, the damage can be repaired, and the individual can be returned to health.

He presented these findings to the University of Tubingen in Germany where he had taught for five years, but without testing or disproving his hypothesis, the board demanded he deny his findings or leave the University. Hamer refused to deny what he had proven scientifically, and his license to practice medicine was withdrawn.

Dr. Hamer believed that the present methods of dealing with cancer were barbarous, cruel and completely unnecessary. "Through the millennia," Dr. Hamer protested, "humanity has more or less consciously known that all diseases ultimately have a psychic origin…It is only modern medicine that has turned our animated beings into a bag full of chemical formulas."

His opinions caused such an uproar in the medical community that he was arrested and sentenced to eighteen months in prison in France. Subsequently, he lived in voluntary exile in Spain until March 2007, when he is said to have moved to Norway. (According to Dr. Hamer, much of the opposition was due to the fact that the person who accidentally killed his son was the Prince of Savoy, the last King of Italy's son.)

To illustrate Dr. Hamer's hypothesis, Marie-Anne asked me to write out a timeline highlighting the traumatic events in my life. "At the onset of an illness, we look for the event tied to a family or personal story. Every cancer or cancer-equivalent ailment develops from a severe, highly acute, dramatic and isolating conflict-occurrence shock that registers simultaneously on three levels: a) in the psyche, b) in the brain, and c) on the organs. If we can discover the location of any one of the levels, the other two can be found and unlocked."

I set about my daunting assignment, convinced it would take the better part of a decade to list every drama in my crazy life, but Marie-Ann assured me only the "main events" were needed, those that happened few months before the illnesses. This would show her the pattern she was looking for; we could fill in additional information as more and more memories began to surface.

The following week I returned, assignment in hand, and Marie-Anne proceeded to create a chart. What she was able to see was that my pattern showed a propensity for both the breast cancer I had 15 years before and the kidney cancer I had just recently dealt with. She explained that the breast cancer, since it was in the left breast, was set into motion by a lack of maternal nurturing; the weakness in the kidney was set into motion at the time of my mother's death and my inheritance snatched out from under me. That conflict-shock produced fear—"of loss of security, loss of landmarks"—in Dr. Hamer's terms, "a collapse of existence," which thrust me out of my safe "liquid" environment onto dry land, which threatened my very existence. The biological connection, according to Dr. Hamer, is that the kidney stops eliminating water, the cells begin to multiply to retain the water, and a tumor forms. When the conflict-shock is resolved, the trauma is neutralized and the biology resumes its normal functioning, often resulting in the disappearance of the symptom. On the other hand, "…if a doctor makes a cancer diagnosis, the patient goes into panic; this panic can result in a new conflict-shock. For example, cancer-fear-panic or mortal-death-panic triggers a new cancer—metastasis—which on the face of it will confirm the doctor's first diagnosis." Dr. Hamer has been able to confirm these discoveries with over 40,000 case studies over a period of 28 years.

There are three stages to Marie-Anne's technique: First, to determine the biological meaning of the symptom and explain to the patient the course of healing. Illness is a meaningful biological reaction of the organism's adaptation for survival. Each cell has stored in its genetic material all biological programs needed for survival and is encoded with each step of these survival programs (commonly called illness) that are activated when facing a life-threatening event. Every specific biological conflict corresponds to a specific biological reaction (symptom). In Nature, nothing appears randomly, everything is (bio)-logical.

The second stage is targeting the conflict-shock, the precise moment of the emotional distress that triggered the conflict. This moment usually occurs a few months before the symptom appears. For a deeper cellular deprogramming," Marie-Anne explains, "we usually need to go back in time to find what we call the programming event—the event with a similar emotional distress that awoke the illness-program without yet activating it. This type of event occurs mostly during childhood." To help the client reach that point Marie-Anne uses tools such as The

Project-sense of the Child, Memorized Biological Cellular Cycles, and Biogenealogy®.

The final step is to transcend the emotional conflict on the cellular level. Marie-Anne uses different techniques such as Bio-NLP (Neuro Languistic Programming applied to Biodecoding®) and Transgenerational techniques, which help to reveal the pattern. The goal is to change the patient's perception of traumatic events in order to neutralize the emotional impact, making it possible for physiological healing to take place.

Other tools are brought into play: one similar to Gestalt therapy, to unlock emotions tied to events in early childhood that have never been resolved; and what I think of as an archaeological dig, to get at memories that have been buried and mummified for years. There is before, there is after. There is now.

Marie-Anne encourages her clients to interrupt the old patterns of thinking and behaving by healing the animalistic fears behind every emotional distress, neutralize them with keen awareness, and instead become an objective observer of one's habitual thoughts in order to make change possible.

This is not easy, it requires discipline and will and an utter passion to heal. "You can't escape from a prison you can't see."

STEPHEN WARD, CHIROPRACTOR

· · · · · · · · · · · ·

THE ANSWERS, MY FRIEND,
LIE NOT IN THE STARS, BUT IN OUR SPINES

Upon entering Dr. Steve's office I am suddenly engulfed in a hug by a giant in a Hawaiian shirt. Bald, smiling, the body of a fullback and the face of an angel, the giant looks at me, his smile broadening. "Hello, beautiful, how's it going today?"

A moment later he's hugging someone else goodbye, and singing out, "Oh, I'm having so much fun today!" Wondering if I've come to the right place, I look around the waiting room and see seven or eight people sitting, chatting and laughing. One of them sits in a vibrating recliner, one is in a neck collar, another in a wheelchair, "I forget why I came in today," a woman laughs, "nothing hurts now."

A slide show of startlingly beautiful photography with quotes from poets, philosophers and anyone who strikes Dr. Steve's fancy plays through a monitor on a table in the corner.

I'm shown to a room with a treatment table, a couple of comfortable chairs, a large desk, with its computer screen facing the room, and on the wall behind the desk, four X-rays up against a light box.

Dr. Steve and I have spoken on the phone so he knows why I've come. My purpose is two-fold: chronic low-back pain and to learn more about his unique practice I've heard so much about. He knows nothing about my health history.

"Have a seat," he says patting the treatment table, "back to me. Let's see what's going on here." As he rubs his huge hands over my neck and shoulders to my sighs of pleasure and relief, he says, "Mmm. Left curvature spine. Now, let's have you lie down, face down." He measures the length of my legs, "Left leg shorter. Gender issues with your mom. You're second-born, right?"

I nod, peering at him. "How would you possibly know that?"

"Dad had heart problems. You have trouble expressing hurt, you keep it inside and rationalize it away. Same with anger."

He stands and looks at me. "You fit the profile. Had you by any chance dealt with some form of cancer in the past?"

I sit up. "*What?* Wait a minute. I get it now. I've walked into a psychic's office by mistake."

Dr. Steve laughs. "No mystery. I ran my hands along your spine—what is called a synchronous test where I test each vertebra to determine what to adjust. I found you have a lower back vertebra out of place and a reversal of the lumbar curve, which I could see just by looking at you. That curve deals with a female parent, and how you learned to deal with hurt."

I'm still baffled. I try to remember where I heard of this man, then it comes to me. A homeopathic doctor I recently met gave him raves, but warned he was "different."

"Your mom learned to deal with hurt through internaliza-tion and denial, and she passed that down to you, which is how you deal with hurtful experiences, through internalization. Whenever you looked to your mom for a lifeline, she'd throw you an anchor. She couldn't help it; it was all she knew how to do. Nothing personal."

I gulp and listen, wide-eyed as he goes on to describe my father and his way of relating to my mother.

"You have a backward curve that indicates the withdrawal of the male parent. Did your dad have any heart issues? If that was an issue with him, that would indicate that he was passive in his life and he would attract a dominant controlling wife."

"How in the world could you possibly know this?"

"I learned this at the feet of my dad who said it's all in the spinal curvature. Over years and years of study, he found that disease, both physical and mental, shows up in a specific spinal curvature pattern. His dad was Dr. Lowell Ward, founder of Spinal Column Stressology (SCS). He was interested in the correlation between spinal curvature and human behavior. He developed a spinal blueprint which he used to study diseased conditions, mental/emotional behaviors and the impact of inherited behavior. For instance, heart disease which shows up as a backward curve of the spine. "My dad would take an X-ray, then he would watch and listen to his patient's story. The patient might say, 'I'm having a heart problem' and my dad would look at the person's X-ray and see what the commonality was between him and another patient with a heart problem. What he found was that among the emotional patterns were patterns of denying one's feelings of hurt.

"He found this by taking measurements on a full spine X-ray

and looking at them on a comparative basis. When one person came in with a particular problem, my dad would make note of it, take the four full spinal X-rays and measure the key angles and spinal landmarks on the spine. When another person came in with the same problem, he'd take a new set of X-rays, mark the measurements, and then take both sets and look for the commonality."

We then talked about cancer. I asked him if he had found a cancer profile.

Dr. Steve explained that he had. "In breast or uterine cancer, typically you'll find left spinal curves, which indicates they have learned to rationalize their hurt. Instead of saying, 'Hey, you're hurting me,' the left curve personality rationalizes, 'Well, they didn't mean that, that's just the way they are.' Instead of expressing their true hurt feelings, they withdraw and deny them. People in left curve operate more in fear."

The chiropractic philosophy is usually a segmental approach to the body. Chiropractic focuses on a segment of the spine and looks for the local pathology—arthritis, disc degeneration, a collapsing lumbar spine. "But when you look at it segmentally you never understand the reason why the pathology occurred, you only understand the result of the pathology.

"What causes disc injury in the lower back is the lumbar curve above deviating backwards, causing a reversal in the normal lumbar curve. The behavior pattern associated with disc injury in the lower back reflects the pattern of a person who takes their hurtful experiences internally. The hurt that we deny is the hurt we wind up feeling in our bodies."

Dr. Steve explained further how he knew my cancer issue was in the past. "The curvature of the spine reveals a healthy defense system; also you did not have a short right leg. When a woman has a short right leg, this is an indication of an immune-compromised state; if it were even shorter, it would indicate a state of exhaustion, which is common in a cancer process. When I see that I refer a patient to a medical doctor."

Dr. Steve's work with boys suffering from Duchenne muscular dystrophy came to national attention when he appeared on the Today Show and on Montel Williams. He began working with these kids in 1990 and has treated over 200 Duchenne patients over the years, many of whom were of necessity in his free program. I was especially interested because of my firsthand experience with a charming and brilliant 12-year-old boy, Alexander, whom I had come to know in Brazil, while researching *The Brazilian Healer with the Kitchen Knife*. Alexander's parents had given up their home and work in Holland to move to Abadiania to be near John of God. In spite of their utter faith that Alexander would be healed, in spite of their prayers and meditations and daily healing sessions with John of God, Alexander only lived another four years—the same age at which most Duchenne kids die. With Dr. Steve's treatments and his unique emotional coaching, his way of reframing the patient's belief that his lifespan is limited, Dr. Steve's kids are living quality lives into their late 20s. I saw a 27-year-old leaving his office who had graduated from college with a major in Criminal Justice. In order to attend classes, he had to take three buses in his wheelchair entirely on his own, there and back. There is a wonderful piece on him on Dr. Steve's website that brought tears when I read it.

· · · · · · · · · · · ·

I was interested to discover that another chiropractor, Dr. Joe Dispenza, author of scientific articles on the close relationship between brain chemistry, neurophysiology, and biology, described a similar process in his book, *Evolve Your Brain*: "Your every thought produces a biochemical reaction in the brain. The brain then releases chemical signals that are transmitted to the body, where they act as messengers to the thought. The thoughts that produce the chemicals in your brain allow the body to *feel* exactly the way you were just *thinking*."

JEANETTE MORRIS
• • • • • • • • • • • •
HORSES AND HUMANS
AND ALL CREATURES IN BETWEEN

There is an ethereal, almost otherworldly quality about Swedish-born Jeanette Morris, who is blond, blue-eyed and fragile in appearance. One soon finds out why. What strikes me is that without exception every one of the healers I have met has had tragedies of some sort in their own lives they had managed to overcome, leaving them with a heightened sensitivity and a gift for healing.

The story of Jeanette's difficult childhood, marked with abandonment and the death of both parents, explains in part her extraordinary gift as a healer. As a child, Jeanette was quiet and withdrawn. "I preferred to communicate silently with animals and the angels who were always around me," she says in a quiet, accented voice.

I met her soon after her arrival here from Sweden. Word had gotten out about her miraculous healing of a horse being stalled in a nearby stable. When I heard that she also heals people and their dogs, cats, snakes, or to borrow from James Herriot's title, All Creatures Great and Small, I wanted to meet her. I made an appointment to see her in her Burbank apartment that she shares with her musician-husband, Kyle, and their 3-year-old daughter, Lilja.

She explains that in order to read the blueprint of a person's body lying on her table, she has to completely leave her own body and enter into the world of her patient's. I lie fully clothed on her table in her office, staring at the bookcase filled with textbooks in Swedish and her collection of artifacts. She asks me if I'd like background music; but, since I have to strain to hear her, I decline. I don't want to miss a word of what she has to tell me.

What she says astounds me. She intuits that I had been dealing with cancer and that it was in one of my organs--kidney, most likely--and that it was now gone. "You have successfully healed the root cause of the cancer; it will not come back."

I ask her how she gets this information. "Your body tells me," she answers simply. Her hands are placed on my feet, then on my legs, knees, head. These are acupressure points that are connected, she explains, to certain organs. Her eyes are closed. She explains she is releasing blocked energy and at the same time increasing the energy flow. By the end of the two-hour session, she has a full picture.

"The blueprint for cancer begins with three factors, all of which build over a long period of time: pH level, stagnated toxins (both environmental and emotional), and a poorly functioning immune system,"

Jeanette holds degrees in phytotherapy (botanical medicine), health care, and in reiki as a Grand Master from a school in Sweden. Her studies also included basic medicine, anatomy, nutrition, sports injuries, energy massage, flower remedies, acupressure, herbal medicine, dog psychology, animal communication. When she completed her studies, she trained with a well-known holistic kinesiologist, Marita Piela, who taught her the use of acupressure, massage, nutrition, and psychology for both animals and humans.

Soon after she arrived in Los Angeles, Jeanette heard about an abandoned Arabian temporarily kept at a nearby stable that was suffering from malnutrition and badly injured hooves. In less than two weeks, Jeanette was able to restore the Arabian to health. Indeed, she learned the horse had been trained in dressage and might now have a new career. She has since healed and rescued other horses.

Soon after I saw Jeanette, Charley seemed sick. She wasn't eating, and she was furiously scratching and biting her skin. Jeanette came to my home and worked on her. It seems Charley had developed a yeast infection, a condition that vets usually treat with steroids and other strong medications. Quietly, Jeanette held her in her arms for an hour or so and suggested some supplements and nutritional changes. "She's okay," she said. "She's just picking up on your stress." I was in the middle of book signings and interviews and yes, I was certainly stressed.

Charley has resumed her duties as my familiar, and I have a new healer to add to my list!

SANDRA CAPELLI, CRANIALSACRO THERAPIST
· · · · · · · · · · · ·
BREATH OF LIFE

Robust, dark-haired, dark-eyed like one of those lusty women in a Fellini movie (she is half Italian, half Portuguese), Sandra arrives with a heavy canvas bag slung over her shoulder. Besides her massage table she's got oils, music (Brazilian's my favorite) and other objects for magical healing. I lay face up fully clothed on the table, Charley occasionally jumping up for a quick massage. For an hour-and-a-half, I give myself to Sandra's gentle rocking and light touch. She explains that she is releasing the restrictions in the craniosacral system to improve the lymphatic flow to the membranes and cerebrospinal fluid that surround and protect the brain and spinal cord. This in turn improves the functioning of the central nervous system.

As I understand it, the natural movements at the skull bones come from the membrane that lines the nervous system structures, namely the brain and spinal cord, which is why the focus is on those membranes, Sandra says, rather than directly on the bones and sutures. Lymphatic drainage is part of her treatment too, a technique that cleanses and improves the immune system.

While Sandra works her magic, I drift off to the beaches of Brazil. I return sans tan but feeling as tall and young and lovely as the girl from Ipanema.

CONTACT INFORMATION

. . . .

Whenever one of my demons rises up and challenges me to a duel, I sound the call to any one of these healers and practitioners. I hear about others from time to time and make it a point to check them out. I will be writing about them in my newsletter, so stay tuned.

. . . .

www.mysticsandhealers.com

www.thirteenthmoonbook.com

Dr. Jim MacKimmie
www.knowingheart.com

Paulo Klikovic
www.pavaoklickovic.com

Melissa Deedon
www.TheAnswerWithin.com

Judith Simon Prager
www.judithprager.com

Dr. Stephen Ward
Long Beach, CA
(562) 420-8884
www.chiroman.com

Ken Kobayashi
www.kenkobayashi.com

Mary Hardy, MD
The Ted Mann
Family Resource Center UCLA
cancerresources@mednet.ucla.edu

Dr. Hans Gruenn
Longevity Center of Los Angeles
(310) 966-9194
www.drgruenn.com

Marie-Anne Boularand
The Biodecoding Institute
Altadena, CA
Tel/Fax (321) 989-2189
www.biodecoding.com

Jeanette Morris
HolisticKinesiologist.com

Sandra Capelli
CranialSacro Therapist
(323) 822-0053
Michael Mohoric
QigongEnergyHealing.com

Bruno Groening
Circle of Friends
www.brunogroening.org

ACKNOWLEDGEMENTS

· · · · · · · · · · · ·

I owe a huge debt to Judith Simon Prager and Harry Youtt, who urged me on and kept a careful eye on every step along the way, and to Babette Sparr, my "sandal lady" who never stopped believing in me; to Mark Robinson for his tireless and loving, technical support; Marcia Horn, president of International Cancer Advocacy Group for her invaluable information and evaluation of medical tests;

I am indebted, too, to Michael Roney, an indefatigable and ever optimistic agent, thanks. I am eternally grateful to Jan Keller, who wields a mean semicolon, for his formidable editing (any stray commas are my fault, not his). My sincere thanks to Celeste Torrens for helping me keep it together with tea and sympathy and words of wisdom; and to friends who walked much of this journey with me: Julie Adams, Margery Nelson, Alex Street, Betty Fussell, who kept reminding me I could; Carol Moss, Lee and Helen Maynard, Chris Rungé for providing puppy love to Charley and additional research to me; Ingrid Watson, Tahdi Blackstone, Jim and Andrea MacKimmie, Sue Terry, Jack

O'Connor for his generous encouragement and support; Bruce Lipton, who was so generous with his time; Terry van Vliet for reading and rereading many drafts; Adam Rodman, Masha Nordbye and Sebastian Toettcher for contributing background music to my healing. Doctors Bryan Baughman, Robert O. Young, and Mary Hardy for their contribution to my research. My thanks, too, to Lucia Colizoli, MD for continually tuning into the heilstrom for me, and to Alicia Papanek for her elegant design.

My abiding gratitude to my son Billy and his wife HJ Paik for Billy and Danny who light up my life on a daily basis; and to my grandsons scattered across the country: AJ, Alec and Owen, and Josh.

Physicist Dan Nelson for sharing his revolutionary discoveries in the field of super-hydrating water and his research in new healing modalities; and to Elliot Ponchek for his stories about our beloved Moses.

And to the best White Coats this side of the rainbow who saw me through the dark days: Doctors Keith Agre, MD, and David Quinn, and Phil Yalowitz, thank you.

SUGGESTED READING

· · · · · · · · · · · · ·

Evolve Your Brain; The Science of Changing Your Mind
Joe Dispenza, D.C. (HCI Communications)

Molecules of Emotion
Candace Pert, PhD. (Scribner 1997)

Anti Cancer; a New Way of Life
by David Servan-Schreiber, MD, PhD (Viking Press)

Journey to Alternity:
Transformational Healing Through Stories and Metaphors,
Judith Simon Prager, PhD (iUniverse)

Verbal First Aid(tm): Help Your Kids Heal From Fear and Pain—
And Come Out Strong
Judith Simon Prager, PhD and Judith Acosta, LISW
(Berkley Books, 2010)

Beating Cancer with Nutrition,
Patrick Quillin (Nutrition Times Press)

The China Study
T. Colin Campbell & Thomas M. Campbell II (Benbella
Publishing)

Presence of Angels: A Healer's Life
J.C. Hugh MacKimmie (Knowing Heart Publishing)

Bruno Groening – Revolution in Medicine
Matthias Kamp, MD (GmbH Publications)

The Biology of Belief:
Unleashing the Power of Consciousness, Matter and Miracles
Bruce Lipton, PhD

Start Where You Are; A Guide to Compassionate Living
Pema Chödödröm (Shambala Classics)

Biology of Belief; Unleashing the Power of Consciousness,
Matter & Miracles
Bruce H. Lipton (Hay House)

And finally for:
Face Lifting By Exercise
Senta Maria Rungé (Allegro Publishing Co.)
www.faceliftingbyexercise.com

· · · · · · · · · · · ·

Book & Cover Design by Alicia Papanek
Illustrations by Marissa Papanek, Aaron Needham & Alicia Papanek
Typefaces used : DIN Next, Adobe Caslon, & Lauren Script
Sandy Johnson Portrait Photography by Paul Reese
Printed in The United States of America

· · · · · · · · · · · ·

8752457R0

Made in the USA
Lexington, KY
27 February 2011